"The game is up for global public health. Richardson delivers a withering critique of a discipline that has too long systematically ignored the real structural and political drivers of disease. If our analysis doesn't account for class, race, and colonial power, then we've missed the point. Fresh, creative, and even tricksteresque—don't miss this book."

—Jason Hickel, University of London; author of *The Divide: Global Inequality from Conquest to Free Markets*

"Far too many of our efforts to achieve equity in health outcomes for everyone everywhere are underpinned by dangerous but unexamined assumptions and premises. Eugene Richardson shows us how to recognize them, take them apart, one by one, and commit them to the dustbin of coloniality where they belong. This book is set to become a prime text for our efforts to decolonize global health."

—Seye Abimbola, University of Sydney; and Editor in Chief, *BMJ Global Health*

"An impressive deconstruction of global health's colonial roots. This fine book is as sophisticated in social theory and history as it is in infectious diseases and medicine. The author doesn't just talk the talk of anthropology, public health, and clinical medicine; he walks the walk, and is as much at home as an ethnographer in West African Ebola settings as in the seminar room discussing postmodern theory, African history, and the imperial background of global health institutions. A telling contribution!"

—Arthur Kleinman, author of *The Soul of Care*

Epidemic Illusions

Epidemic Illusions

On the Coloniality of Global Public Health

Eugene T. Richardson

Foreword by Paul Farmer

The MIT Press
Cambridge, Massachusetts
London, England

This book was set in ITC Stone Serif Std and ITC Stone Sans Std by New Best-set Typesetters Ltd. Printed and bound in the United States of America.

Library of Congress Cataloging-in-Publication Data

Names: Richardson, Eugene T., author.
Title: Epidemic illusions : on the coloniality of global public health / Eugene T. Richardson ; foreword by Paul Farmer.
Description: Cambridge, Massachusetts : The MIT Press, [2020] | Includes bibliographical references and index.
Identifiers: LCCN 2020011240 | ISBN 9780262045605 (paperback)
Subjects: MESH: Epidemics | Global Health | Colonialism | Anthropology | Africa
Classification: LCC RA651 | NLM WA 105 | DDC 614.4—dc23
LC record available at https://lccn.loc.gov/2020011240

10 9 8 7 6 5 4 3

To my parents

Contents

Foreword: Gramsci, but More Pragmatic

> One of the great challenges of any social movement is to develop new vocabularies.
> —Angela Y. Davis, "Marcuse's Legacies"

Of a raft of new publications about Ebola, *Epidemic Illusions* is the most important I've read to date. That's because Eugene Richardson is asking the key questions of the day: What do racism and diverse forms of belittlement and exclusion have to do with epidemics? How do we best understand their progress and unequal toll? How are these virulent outlooks built into public health and academic discourses?

These questions aren't new ones. They've been around for centuries and more, but are being asked, here, by a physician-anthropologist at a time when many without such specialized training are posing them vehemently. Richardson's book appears as the world is covered—unevenly, as ever with pandemics—by a new disease, and by an awakening to the perils of an old pathology, his nation's oldest one: racism has enjoyed a long run in the United States, where neither public health nor epidemiology, argues Richardson, recognize their collusion in reproducing it. But this is a global pathology, as is the coloniality he dissects. These problems persist both here and there, with "there" meaning (in this book) the former colonies. Which is to say, the Majority World.

For years, I've argued that the discipline of *global health equity* represents a sharp break with colonial medicine. But I find Richardson presents a more compelling, if less materialist, argument. He doesn't mince words in arguing that, "as an apparatus of *coloniality*, Public Health *manages* (as a profession) and *maintains* (as an academic discipline) global health inequity." There are several grammatical and formatting qualifiers throughout the book, including capital letters and italics, but these seem to be references, and there are many, to a previous century's logics and styles. He proposes novel connections, if novelty is defined as an application of old ideas and insights to new epidemics: drawing on Mikhail Bakhtin, for example, Richardson proposes a sort of textual "carnivalization" in order "to unsettle webs of meaning and power in global health." This, without question, he has done.

Carnivalization works its way into most pages of this book, even its most somber ones. Richardson's prose is often carnivalesque, but he wastes no time getting serious business out of the way. He acknowledges white privilege—"You are a colonizer through and through. You can feel it in your bones, which have never known stunting. It courses through your veins, through which malaria never has. Every fiber of your being has been nurtured by centuries of predatory accumulation"—even as he sends up his own training in anthropology, which he turns on the strange culture of "experts" in public health and epidemiology. At the World Health Organization, for example, Richardson the anthropologist "was able to establish sufficient rapport to examine their relics and join their rituals."

Is this a joke? An inside joke? A philosophical exercise divorced, as so many of them are, from the real-world challenges of countering epidemic disease? It's not a joke. ("When thousands of people start bleeding out of their mouths and eyes," as Richardson quotes in introducing Ebola as a theme, "sometimes it's best to take a step back and see where it's all going.") With rare exceptions, global health inequality—and the noxious ideologies that have been the blueprint for it—have marred most colonial and postcolonial efforts to address epidemic disease. In a time when more and more people make the connection between pandemics and social inequality, with structural racism front and center, our flawed analyses of outbreaks are too often a form of status quo propaganda, and a mediocre one at that. For those outside of these circles and facing a heightened threat from such epidemics, it's not funny at all.

If the text of *Epidemic Illusions* is sometimes marked by japery, it's more marked by subtlety. Can one operate as an effective critic of modernity while using its terms of reference? Borrowing from Edward Said, Richardson approaches global public health as a form Orientalism—in short, aiming to exhibit the discipline of epidemiology as a discursive space amenable to cultural criticism. Some of its practitioners, he writes, "have had their moral outlooks stunted by coloniality." In these pages, a long riff about an arcane Ebola debate is often followed by devastating empirical insight about how such discourse is reflected in the stunted analyses in much research, writing, and sundry official commentary.

It can be a most trenchant critique. Why, Richardson asks, is there so much attention to stigma, often parsed as a local and cultural response to noxious events, but insufficient attention to structural racism? Why is he able to find, logging on to PubMed, over 5,000 articles about AIDS and "stigma," while there are only 200 or so about HIV and racism? Is it because the term "stigma" is often used, in practice and sometimes in theory, to stunt our understanding of the forces promoting suffering among the afflicted, diverting our attention to their alleged cultural or cognitive deficiencies, whereas exploring racism, especially structural racism, turns our attention instead to power—particularly the power of extractive colonial rule and white supremacy, and the varied regimes of coloniality they spawned?

2.

As Covid-19 slowed or halted much of everyday social life, and especially since the murder of George Floyd, a broader audience turned tardily to questions that have captured Gene Richardson's attention for most of the past two decades. I'd like to introduce this book by introducing him.

I got to know Richardson in 2014 in a makeshift Ebola Treatment Unit, or ETU, at the height of Sierra Leone's epidemic. After subsequent years of working and writing with him, I knew this book would be informed by a profound knowledge of epidemics, extensive personal experience in responding to them in West Africa and elsewhere, and an enduring commitment to pragmatic solidarity. What I didn't expect was the degree to which *Epidemic Illusions* would engage in logical and conceptual debates, and even philosophical ones. Richardson, I thought in reading an early version of his book, is like Gramsci but more pragmatic (in the Rortian sense). And while Gramsci was an organizer, Richardson chose tending to the sick as his praxis.

He was born to an upwardly mobile family in a New Jersey suburb in 1976 and grew up in Florida. His engagement in health and social justice wasn't sure back then—"I revered Nixon because Alex P. Keaton did," he said slyly when I asked about his childhood—but medicine, not politics, was the profession to which he aspired. As an undergraduate at Duke University, he majored in biology as a pre-med and, shortly after graduating, traveled to Cape Town, South Africa, to continue studies in anthropology and generally prolong his errant learning. But he "didn't like what was going on there, as the university was still hypercolonized. Rhodes still sat demonically in front of the place, but the movement to fell him was still sixteen years away."

Something had happened, clearly, between venerating Nixon and execrating Rhodes. Richardson next applied to a master's program in anthropology in Sydney, Australia. Upon arrival, he discovered that the program in anthropology was closing. "What else you got?" he says he asked. "Asian studies, Eastern philosophy, ancient Chinese Buddhism?" So he surfed and read omnivorously, heading next for China (where he ended up in, of all places, Wuhan) and then for another semester-long program in India, where he played cricket with Tibetan refugees and furthered his studies of esoteric Buddhist philosophy. On a hiking trip in Nepal, Richardson was stricken with hepatitis E. When his parents came to collect their son, they found him "terrifically jaundiced" and bought him a return ticket the next day.

Back in Florida, Richardson "recovered, got a job at a record store and on a radio show, and took oceanography classes." His interest in "Eastern" thought continued unabated, and he decided to go next to the University of Hawaii to pursue graduate studies on the topic, but was unsure which discipline to work in. His reading led him also to studies of how social inequalities, including racism, got in the body. And his interest in health and social justice, and in pragmatic solidarity, didn't wither either. These fused with the relational view of phenomena he had come to embrace, motivating his application to medical school—against the recommendations of his previous Buddhist teachers, who said he would destroy all he had learned. Unconvinced, he ended up taking a master's in tropical medicine. He organized a practicum in Peru, where he had his first, if abortive, contact with Partners In Health, the NGO we both work with. ("I got fired after a month for being obnoxious—basically I wanted to join the teachers' protests in Lima instead of doing the hard work of clinical research, tedious work I now know saves lives" was how Richardson put it. I had no idea he'd worked with us before the West African Ebola outbreak.) Aborting his master's a semester shy of graduating, he took up a volunteer position with Doctors Without Borders, where he spent five months in strife-racked Sudan, supervising the clinical lab at a field hospital.

It was in Sudan, Richardson said, that he saw how even the best-intentioned humanitarian efforts could unwittingly serve imperial ends. He returned to the United States to attend medical school in New York City, at Cornell. By then, it seems to me, Richardson was clearly enough on his current path, even if the Upper East Side was a tough proving ground for global health equity. He took a year off from medical school, returning to South Africa at a time when global health policy fights centered less on access to therapy—those battles were drawing to a close, even in the country with the world's largest number of HIV infections—than on standards of care, which came to be one of the subjects on which he would take a repeated and coherent stand.

The standard-of-care issues were anything but carnivalesque. At the outset of the antiviral era, battles in Pretoria and other cities turned on what to do to prevent transmission from mother to child during breastfeeding. Exclusive breastfeeding remained a public health recommendation for HIV-positive African mothers, but not for those who delivered infants in Geneva, Washington, or Boston, for example. The alternative recommended to the affluent world, formula feeding, was deemed by public health experts *not* to be cost-effective, sustainable, culturally appropriate, or even feasible. Lack of ready access to the wherewithal to prepare formula—running water, a stove or a fire, clean receptacles—was readily documented in the villages and neighborhoods to which many mothers delivering in public hospitals across the continent returned. But couldn't this wherewithal be found?

This and related dilemmas led Richardson to conclude that he needed "to become better versed in the structural determinants of health and illness." Upon graduation from medical school, in 2009, he went to Stanford to pursue clinical training in internal medicine and infectious disease—to become a professional pragmatist—and a doctoral degree in anthropology. He was soon dividing his time between HIV clinic and classes in northern California. He did much of his doctoral research in South Africa, focusing on AIDS and tuberculosis, the two leading killers there. In South Africa, he turned to understanding pathogenic social forces—ranging from forced removals and labor migration to gender inequality and persistent post-apartheid racism—and how these might best be mitigated in efforts to slow epidemics and to deliver good care to those sickened during them. "I focused on structural violence," he explained, "since there are approximately twelve thousand HIV investigators in South

Africa looking at stigma, culture, psychology, local knowledge, and cognition; there seemed to be even more looking at cost-effectiveness of this or that narrowly focused intervention."

I've underlined Gene Richardson's pragmatism (both philosophically and as praxis) in part because those focusing on structural determinants are sometimes dismissed as being "impractical," and in part because I met him shortly after this stage of his career, at the close of his doctoral and clinical training. The outbreak of Ebola that began in Guinea at the close of 2013 was first identified as such a few months later. He had maintained his ties with Doctors Without Borders and volunteered for service, ending up in the town of Kailahun, in eastern Sierra Leone—leveled by war a decade previously and now home to an explosive Ebola epidemic. The epidemic was heading westward to the large cities on the coast of Upper West Africa; it was an awful time. Since that time is covered in this book, it won't be covered here, even though Richardson's narrative is tucked in between carnivalized asides about the logics of cost-effectiveness and clinical nihilism: Ebola, we heard, is too operose to treat properly in such settings.

After arguments about whether or not intravenous fluids could be used to resuscitate dehydrated Ebola patients in Kailahun, Richardson applied for the Ebola work being conducted by Partners In Health, an organization he works with to this day from Harvard Medical School.

3.

It wasn't until after he joined our faculty that Gene Richardson traveled to the eastern Democratic Republic of the Congo, where he and several of our colleagues helped to respond to another large outbreak of Ebola. At the risk of repeating myself, he is a thoroughgoing pragmatist, just the sort of person you'd want by your side in the midst of an epidemic.

There are other reasons to be enamored of, and instructed by, *Epidemic Illusions*. You will love not only its playfulness; you will love its devotions. Richardson makes reference to a bit of verse by Bertolt Brecht, the German playwright who brought us *Mother Courage*. In his famous "A Worker's Speech to a Doctor," Brecht poses the following questions:

> When we visit you
> Our clothes are ripped and torn
> And you listen all over our naked body.
> As to the cause of our illness
> A glance at our rags would be more
> Revealing. One and the same cause wears out
> Our bodies and our clothes.
>
> The pain in our shoulder comes
> You say, from the damp; and this is also the cause
> Of the patch on the apartment wall.
> So tell us then:
> Where does the damp come from?
>
> Too much work and too little food
> Make us weak and scrawny.
> Your prescription says:
> Put on more weight.
> You might as well tell a fish
> Go climb a tree
>
> How much time can you give us?
> We see: one carpet in your flat costs
> The fees you take from
> Five thousand consultations

> You'll no doubt protest
> Your innocence. The damp patch
> On the wall of our apartments
> Tells the same story.

Richardson assumes, throughout this book, a familiarity with colonial and postcolonial debates about class, caste, and race, and he also assumes his reader might know Brecht, which is why the physician-anthropologist offers an ersatz tribute to Brecht in a book about standards of care for those at the bottom of the global totem pole:

> When we come to you
> With hemorrhagic fever
> And you isolate us with only ORS,
> As to the cause of our illness
> An exploration of the kimberlite pipe
> Would tell you more. It is the same reason
> We don't polish or cut our diamonds here.
>
> The untreated hypovolemic shock comes,
> You say, from an underdeveloped health infrastructure,
> And this is also the reason
> That 1 in 17 of our mothers will die in childbirth.
> So tell us:
> Where does this underdevelopment come from?

This is certainly not a joke, nor is any of the rest of *Epidemic Illusions*. It's a book about many things—Ebola, for sure, but also coloniality, racism, and the insidious role Northern institutions play (through cultural hegemony) in perpetuating global health inequities—which is one of the reasons I've compared Richardson to Gramsci. When asked why he chose to focus in this book on Ebola, rather than the other plagues he's battled, Richardson's answer managed to span the clinical and the epistemological:

It just so happens to be a disease I'm familiar with clinically. When you're working in an ETU every day, participant-observation doesn't mean sitting in the green zone conducting an ethnography of the place. That's a different form of knowledge production. You have to pitch in. But I'm arguing here that the way the Global North parses epidemics and related phenomena is not a value-neutral act contributing to some growing body of shared knowledge. Too often, and despite what epidemiologists would have you believe, this parsing is a form of symbolic power, that is, the ability to impose ways of understanding suffering—often on the sufferers themselves. Acts of epistemic violence are part of the injustice people face every day.

Eugene Richardson's commitment to "democratizing knowledge" in settings of severe material deprivation is reason alone to return to this slim volume in the coming years. Another lies in his consideration of reparations and repair—yet another conversation he is leading within academic medicine. This will be, even in these rarefied circles, a tough one. In the meantime, let this book serve as a means of developing new vocabularies and stoking debates, for no social movement can thrive without them.

Paul Farmer

Preface

This endeavor, to be consistent in its methodologically relation-
ist aspirations, must necessarily admit that no single author was
responsible for its product. Moreover, no network-reflexive (as
opposed to self-reflexive) pseudomonograph worth its salt can
begin without describing the matrix of relationships within
which it is embedded.

Accordingly, the EUGENE T. RICHARDSON (ETR) that bedecks
the title page is the mere alphabetical representation of a single node in a vast, interconnected net of support, mentoring,
toleration, encouragement, inspiration, and generosity. Other
nodes could be labeled ANNA RICHARDSON (любимая) or PAUL
FARMER or JAMES HOLLAND JONES or WIILIAM H. DURHAM
or DONNALEE RICHARDSON or EUGENE T. RICHARDSON III
or EUGENE T. RICHARDSON II or EUGENE T. RICHARDSON I or
BRIAN P. RICHARDSON or NICOLE K. RICHARDSON or BEVERLY
TERRELL or GREG C. MINDEL or ANDREW R. ZOLOPA or JULIE
PARSONNET or MICHELE BARRY or KELLEY M. SKEFF or KIM
MNUSKIN or IRINA ABRAMSON or PARTNERS IN HEALTH or
@UGHE or SHEILA DAVIS or JOEL MUBILIGI or PETER DROBAC
or IMANA or MONICA LEE or MATTHEW HORNING or SEAN
COLLINS or TANAYA SHREE or CHRISTINE SAVAGE or ANTHONY

OGEDEGBE or OLIVER T. FEIN or EVAN WHITFIELD or KEVIN
LOCHNER or CHRISTOPHER HURLEY or IAN CROZIER or DENEB
PELLETIER or MAMA LUZ or ADIA BENTON or ANGELA GAR-
CIA or TANYA MARIE LUHRMANN or JOÃO BIEHL or NANCY
KASS or CATHERINE PANTER-BRICK or KEARSLEY STEWART or
NANCY SCHEPER-HUGHES or J. DANIEL KELLY or CASEY BAR-
BARO or GRANT SISLER or RAJAIE BATNIJI or ROBIN WOOD or
LINDA-GAIL BEKKER or CHRIS BEYRER or DANIEL BAUSCH or
MOSOKA P. FALLAH or RICHARD HORTON or TRAVIS C. PORCO
or DANIEL R. KURITZKES or PAUL E. SAX or SIGAL YAWETZ or
JOSEPH RHATIGAN or STEPHEN KAHN or ARTHUR KLEINMAN
or ANNE BECKER or MEGAN B. MURRAY or SALMAAN KESHAV-
JEE or MERCEDES BECERRA or SCOTT PODOLSKY or JOE GONE
or DAVID S. JONES or SETH HOLMES or BYRON GOOD or
MARY-JO DELVECCHIO GOOD or DIDIER FASSIN or WILLIAM
A. DARITY, JR. or KIRSTEN MULLEN or MAXINE BURKETT or
SIR HILARY BECKLES or GEORGES NZONGOLA-NTALAJA or LIE-
POLLO LEBOHANG PHEKO or SUNNEVA GILMORE or CLARA
SANDOVAL or SONJA KLINSKY or SUKHADEO THORAT or AMIT
THORAT or MAGDA MATACHE or BETSY MCKAY or ICHIRO
KAWACHI or JOIA MUKHERJEE or EMMANUEL AKYEAMPONG
or @AFRICAHARVARD or SEIJI YAMADA or JULIE AKE or DAVID
BRETT-MAJOR or CARROLLWOOD VILLAGE SWIM TEAM or
JIM KELLY or ISHAAN DESAI or RAPHAEL FRANKFURTER or LEE
WORDEN or TIM MCGINNIS or AMRAPALI MAITRA or JAKE
ROSENBERG or JON SHAFFER or AMIR MOHAREB or SAM VIDAL
or VINCENT LIN or CAMERON NUTT or ELSIE KARMBOR-
BALLAH or ODELL KUMEH or NTOMBIFUTHI DENNIS or
MARISE KEREHI STUART or ALUSINE DUMBUYA or MICHAEL
DRASHER or MARTA LADO or YUSUPHA DIBBA or BARTHAL-
OMEW WILSON or JAKE MILLER or JASON SILVERSTEIN or

JENNIFER PUCCETTI or KATHERINE KRALIEVITS or LIBBY HIGGS or SHEILA JASANOFF or JEAN COMAROFF or MARTHA LINCOLN or JASON HICKEL or @DUKEDECOLONIZE or SEYE ABIMBOLA or SANJOY BHATTACHARYA or MADHU PAI or MARY BASSETT or JOHN NKENGASONG or SMIT CHITRE or ISADORE NABI or JONATHAN ABRAHAM or JONATHAN MORI or MICHAEL M. J. FISCHER or MOMIN MALIK or MATTHEW BROWNE or ANNE-MARIE BONO or MATTHEW ABBATE or MIT PRESS or GEORGE Q. DALEY or AGNES BINAGWAHO or ABEBE BEKELE or JONATHAN LASCHER or MOHAMED B. BARRIE or KIEREN J. RICHARDSON or BENJAMIN LAY (figure 1).

This node (ETR) shares a network ambition to understand how social, political economic, and cultural factors influence disease distribution, with the twin goals of epistemic reconstitution and improvement of human well-being.

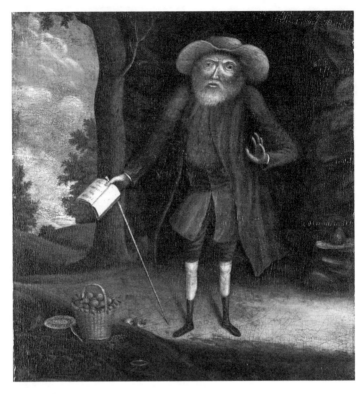

Figure 1
Benjamin Lay: an 18th-century Quaker dwarf polemicist and revolution-
ary abolitionist. (M. Rediker, "You'll Never Be as Radical as This 18th-
Century Quaker Dwarf," *New York Times*, August 12, 2017.)

What then is truth? A mobile army of metaphors, metonyms, and anthropomorphisms—in short, a sum of human relations which have been enhanced, transposed, and embellished poetically and rhetorically, and which after long use seem firm, canonical, and obligatory to a people: <u>truths are illusions about which one has forgotten that this is what they are</u>; metaphors which are worn out and without sensuous power; coins which have lost their pictures and now matter only as metal, no longer as coins.

—Friedrich Nietzsche, *On Truth and Lie in an Extra-Moral Sense* (1873)

Part I
Carnivalization (карнавализация)

The thesis of this book is simple: The continuation of disproportionate amounts of suffering and death from infectious diseases in the Global South is not the result of an intractable problem thwarting our best efforts to prevent and cure disease; we have the means.[1] However, as an apparatus of *coloniality*,[2] Public Health *manages* (as a profession) and *maintains* (as an academic enterprise) global health inequity.[3] It does this through "bourgeois empiricist" models of disease causation,[4] which serve protected affluence (i.e., the possessing classes) by uncritically reifying inequitable social relations in the modern/colonial matrix of power,[5] making them appear commonsensical[6] or elevating them to unchangeable facts.[7]

In order to demonstrate this, I employ what the Russian linguist Mikhail Bakhtin called *carnivalization* (карнавализация).[8] Carnivalized discourse is an approach that dethrones dominant ways of thinking.[9] Much like the medieval festivals from which Bakhtin derived the term (figure 2), where the sacred/profane and sublime/ridiculous would commingle to subvert hierarchies, the following pseudomonograph uses a carnivalesque approach to unsettle webs of meaning and power in global health. Instead

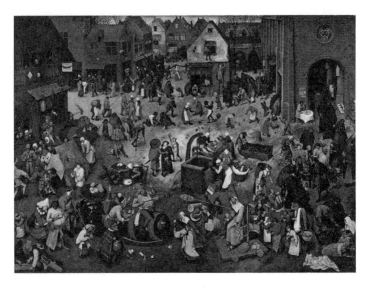

Figure 2
Pieter Bruegel the Elder, *The Fight between Carnival and Lent* (1559).
Kunsthistorisches Museum, Vienna.

of relying on ethnographic description, statistical analysis, rational argument, and other rhetorical apparatuses used to make a text persuasive, this work intends to destabilize and question hegemonic modes of knowing—while imagining alternatives.

Introduction
Pr [Global Health Equity | Coloniality]ⁱ

Hey, this is tough! / Hey, this is tough! / Our soul in a bottle / This
    is tough!
We have to speak like these people / We have to see like these people
    / We have to listen like these people / We have to look like these
    people
When will we arrive / When will we take a stand / My friends this
    is tough!

"Nanm Nan Boutey" (Soul in a Bottle) by the Haitian group
Boukman Eksperyans

Coloniality can be described as the matrix of power relations
that persistently manifests transnationally and intersubjectively
despite a former colony's achievement of nationhood. As a conceptual apparatus, "coloniality" attempts to capture the racial,
political economic, social, epistemological, linguistic, and gen-
dered hierarchical orders imposed by European colonialism
that transcended "decolonization" and continue to oppress in

---

i Statistical notation which translates to "What is the probability of
global health equity in the setting of coloniality?" By the time you reach
the Afterword, you should have an answer.

accordance with the needs of pan-capital (i.e., economic[1] *and* cultural/symbolic[2]) accumulation.[3] Examples of these orders include institutionalized racism,[ii][4] religious discrimination, economic exploitation and architected underdevelopment,[5] control of gender and sexuality,[6] and dominion over subjectivity and knowledge.[7]

My ideas on the coloniality of global public health come from engagements as a privilege-exerciser (white upper-middle-class male settler-colonist)[8] in the Global South and its spigots in the Global North.[iii] Through the various guises of physician, anthropologxxx,[iv][9] researcher, consultant, intern, student, and all-around *mujahid*,[v] I have struggled to understand the causes of epidemics, while aiming to care for groups of people affected by them. I have also wrestled with the "perfect, genuine, complete, crystalline"[vi] inventiveness of authors like Kwame Nkrumah, Frantz Fanon, Edward Said, Toni Morrison, and Paul Farmer—to name but a few—and so my ideas are not "my" ideas[10] per se, but rather a form of network dialogue.

---

ii As the Cameroonian philosopher Achille Mbembe writes, "Our critique of modernity will remain incomplete if we fail to grasp that the coming of modernity coincided with the appearance of the principle of race and the latter's slow transformation into the privileged matrix for techniques of domination, yesterday as today." A. Mbembe, *Critique of Black Reason* (Durham: Duke University Press, 2017).

iii Spigot is defined here as a municipal area (e.g., London, New York, Beijing, Geneva, etc.) where illicit financial flows from the Global South are funneled.

iv Darcy Ribeiro has described the anthropologist as one who is based in the location of the studying object and the anthropologian (*antropologador*) as one who is based in the object of study. D. Ribeiro, *Las Americas y la civilización* (Buenos Aires: Centro Editor de América Latina, 1969).

v مجاهد (Arabic for "struggler").

vi Colonel Kurtz in *Apocalypse Now* (1979).

To paraphrase the artificial intelligence philosopher Philip Agre, "So here I was in the middle of the [global public health world] . . . and yet, day by day, it started to seem insane. This is what I do: I get myself trapped inside of things that seem insane."[11] Insane experience that will be drawn on in the following chapters (i.e., redescriptions) include working with Doctors Without Borders on a leishmania epidemic in the Sudan; with the Desmond Tutu HIV Foundation on HIV/TB in southern Africa; with Partners in Health and the National Institutes of Health on Ebola in West Africa; with the World Bank on HIV prevention in Swaziland; with the World Health Organization on Ebola in the Democratic Republic of the Congo; with the Islamic Medical Association of America on diphtheria among the Rohingya in Bangladesh; and with the Africa CDC on COVID-19.

But the biggest epidemic I have encountered, and the one I struggle most with in this book, is an epidemic of illusions—an epidemic propagated by the coloniality of knowledge production: What are the mechanisms in public health science—in particular, epidemiology—that enable groups to sanction one account of disease causation over another, that is, to achieve monopolies on truth (figure 3)?[12] How do such groups achieve the authoritative status to set public health agendas? And how do their views become reified as common sense, such that other perspectives are marginalized? By engaging with theories of symbolic violence and the coloniality of power, I probe the *illusiveness* of these ways of parsing health phenomena that hold a lock on the imaginations of the public, decision makers, planners, students, and scientists.[13]

*   *   *

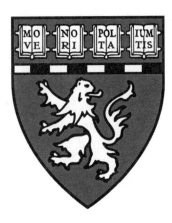

Figure 3
Revised Harvard shield. (Translation from Latin: "Monopoly on Truth.")

Michel Foucault has written:

> Truth is a thing of this world: it is produced only by virtue of multiple forms of constraint. And it induces regular effects of power. Each society has its regime of truth [episteme], its "general politics" of truth: that is, the types of discourse which it accepts and makes function as true; the mechanisms and instances which enable one to distinguish true and false statements, the means by which each is sanctioned; the techniques and procedures accorded value in the acquisition of truth; the status of those who are charged with saying what counts as true.[15]

For simplicity's sake, one could dichotomize regimes of truth into a Have-isteme and a Havenot-isteme. As the sociologist Charles Mills has taught, "if exploitative socioeconomic relations are indeed foundational to the social order, then this is likely to have a fundamental shaping effect on social ideation."[16] The contemporary social "sciences," including economics, political science, sociology, and epidemiology, are epistemic communities that have been configured in a milieu of protected affluence. In the pages ahead, I aim to demonstrate the ways that exploitative socioeconomic relations have been fundamental to shaping how the discipline of epidemiology—in Have-istemic fashion—parses, categorizes, and explains how populations get sick.[vii] I hope to contrast this with examples of Havenot-istemic knowledge production—that it, subjugated ways of interpreting phenomena that do not become hegemonic, owing to the social position of their creators and their often destabilizing ramifications for global elites.

Q: What is an epistemic community?

A: The political scientist Peter Haas defines epistemic community as "a network of professionals with recognized expertise and competence in a particular domain and an authoritative claim to policy-relevant knowledge within that domain or issue-area. Although an epistemic community may consist of professionals from a variety of disciplines and backgrounds, they have (1) a shared set of normative and principled beliefs, which provide a value-based rationale for the social action of community members; (2) shared causal beliefs, which are derived from their analysis of practices leading or contributing to a central set of problems in their domain and which then serve as the basis for elucidating the multiple linkages between possible policy actions and desired outcomes; (3) shared notions of validity—that is, intersubjective, internally defined criteria for weighing and validating knowledge in the domain of their expertise; and (4) a common policy enterprise—that is, a set of common practices associated with a set of problems to which their professional competence is directed, presumably out of the conviction that human welfare will be enhanced as a consequence."[14] Throughout this book, I elevate all idea-sharing groups to the status of epistemic community.

---

vii According to Luc Boltanksi, exploitation "refers to the way that a small number of people make use of differentials (which can be very diverse in kind) in order to extract a profit at the expense of the great majority." L. Boltanski, *On Critique: A Sociology of Emancipation* (Cambridge: Polity, 2011).

Points of Departure

The coloniality of global health praxis has been explored in its various aspects: Meredith Turshen has probed the ideological distortions in contemporary understandings of public health phenomena;[17] Johanna Crane has investigated how global health research partnerships may paradoxically benefit from the very inequalities they aspire to redress;[18] Didier Fassin has traced a moral paradigm (humanitarianism) in which suffering and compassion have come to displace a politics of rights and justice;[19] drawing on Aimé Césaire and Walter Rodney among others, Jason Hickel has shown how development and aid occult the patterns of extraction that are actively causing impoverishment of the Global South;[20] Vincanne Adams and others have theorized the means by which quantitative metrics and their exaggerated precision obscure a range of political phenomena;[21] Adriana Petryna and João Biehl have championed subaltern narratives of health phenomena as a counterbalance to the generation of certainties and foreclosures by epidemiology and other disciplines;[22] William Easterly has exposed the technocratic illusion, which holds that poverty results from a shortage of expertise, whereas it is really about a shortage of rights;[23] Ruha Benjamin has grappled with the means by which science and technology reproduce lethal strains of inequity;[24] Richard Rottenburg has postulated that it becomes difficult to distinguish humanitarian emergencies from chronic poverty when the securing of health is defined as the deployment of biomedicine;[25] Margaret Lock and Vinh-Kim Nguyen have problematized the ontological status of the human body in health and illness;[26] Salmaan Keshavjee has demonstrated how international nongovernmental organizations (NGOs) serve as "transplanting mecha neoliberal ideologies";[27] Richard Horton, Seye Abimbola, a... Madhu Pai have highlighted the contribution of medical journals to colonial interests;[28] Adia Benton has revealed the pathogenic racial legacies of social science inquiry;[29] Sarah Hodges has shown how the "turning away from analyses of power in history-writing leads to scholarship that reproduces rather than critiques globalization";[30] Sam Dubal has challenged normative discourses about the concept of "humanity";[31] and the Humanitarian Women's Network has documented gender discrimination and abuse in the global health workspace.[32] The list goes on.

This book aims to add to the above analyses by exploring the coloniality of global public health science, in particular the discipline of epidemiology. It is my contention that epidemiology—and its growing methodological hegemony in the form of Big Data and causal inference—functions as an ideological apparatus of protected affluence disguised as objective inquiry.[33] Here I define protected affluence[viii] as the set of human networks with greater access to forms of pan-capital, which then manifest as barriers to the fulfillment of fundamental human needs[34] for those without such access.

While recognizing the devastating impact of material deprivation on the health of populations, this book responds to Boaventura de Sousa Santos's claim that global social injustice is

---

viii Jaime Breilh refers to the phenomenon as an "armed form of structural greed." J. Breilh, "Latin American Critical ('Social') Epidemiology: New Settings for an Old Dream," *International Journal of Epidemiology* 37 (2008): 745–750.

by and large epistemological injustice and that there can be no global social justice without addressing symbolic violence.[35] It is my non-novel hypothesis that breaking up the Global North's monopoly on truth will transform global health by transforming its representations.

A Note on Method

> Despite the celebration of decolonization as a milestone in African history of liberation, Africa has not managed to free itself from epistemological colonization, inscribed on the continent and its people by mission and secular schools, religious denominations, and other institutions that carried western cultural imperialism.
>
> —Sabelo J. Ndlovu-Gatsheni, *Coloniality of Power in Postcolonial Africa* (2013)

I first learned about neocolonialism and the critique of development from James Ferguson's *The Anti-Politics Machine* (1990/1994), yet imagine my surprise when I later read most of the ideas it contains (minus the Foucauldian spin) in Kwame Nkrumah's *Neo-colonialism, the Last Stage of Imperialism* (1965), written over 20 years earlier (and not even cited by Ferguson). Once I observed how coloniality permeates even the most ostensibly progressive echelons of academia—where privileged scholars appropriate the intellectual property (IP) of thinkers from the Global South and gentrify it (*The Anti-Politics Machine* has been cited over 8,000 times; *Neo-colonialism* less than a quarter of that total)—I began to recognize it in global health praxis.[ix]

---

ix To slightly misquote Naughty by Nature: "Who's down with OPIP? Yeah, you know me!"

Q: What is postcolonial thinking?

A: "Postcolonial thought is not an anti-European thought. On the contrary, it's the product of the encounter between Europe and the worlds it once made into its distant possessions. In showing how the colonial and imperial experience has been codified in representations, divisions between disciplines, their methodologies and their objects, it invites us to undertake an alternative reading of our common modernity."[36]

It "has thus often worked to destabilize, or at least challenge, the assumption that Western knowledge is objective, authoritative and universally applicable."[37]

The following chapters are based on years of engaged participant observation as an anthropologian in the following institutions: (1) classrooms in American schools of public health, where I acquired competency in statistical methods and the programming languages of EpidemiologySpeak[38] and scrutinized how future global health professionals were "socialized for scarcity"[39] via the inculcation of conservative epistemologies; (2) the World Health Organization and World Bank, where I worked as a consultant; and (3) the frontlines of international nongovernmental-organization efforts to combat Ebola, HIV, tuberculosis, visceral leishmaniasis, diphtheria, and COVID-19.[x] In preparing this book, I have triangulated these accumulated experiential data with the "social science literature" and processed them with Fanonian algorithms to generate a series

---

x In many ways, my study of global public health "has been an attempt to inventory the traces upon me" of a privileged position in the modern/colonial matrix of power. See E. W. Said, *Orientalism* (New York: Vintage, 1979).

of postcolonial heuristics. In some instances, my method is to focus on journal publications, to read them first as great products of the epidemiologic "imagination, and then to show them as part of the relationship between culture and empire."[40] In other instances, I give new expression to the depredation my privilege is based on by plundering a variety of academic disciplines and knowledge ecologies for ways of redescribing social phenomena.

Q: What are heuristics?

A: A heuristic device is "any procedure which involves the use of an artificial construct to assist in the exploration of social phenomena."[41]

Something Is Rotten in the State of Global Health

This book starts from the premise that those who would be convinced by the coupling of compelling empirical evidence with moral arguments à la Paul Farmer[42] have already been convinced. Hence, I have chosen to approach the topics heuristically, rather than via linear argument or conventional ethnography[xi][43]— modes of thinking and writing that are themselves relics of coloniality. For those global health practitioners who have not been convinced, I write à la Edward Said with two ends in mind:[44] (1) to present their intellectual categories in potentially novel fashion (i.e., to jar otherwise opaque relationships into focus);

---

xi However, what follows is ethnographic in the sense that it is based on a "study of social interactions, behaviors, and perceptions that occur within" the tribe of global public health.

and (2) to critique[xii]—with the aim of assembling rather than debunking[45]—the often unquestioned assumptions on which their work for the most part depends. For my colleagues in the so-called Third World / Global South, I express my gratitude up front for their accompanying my unlearning of what Raymond Williams has called "the inherent dominative mode."[46] My aim is not to represent their experience of epistemic violence, but rather to struggle with global health theory and praxis and say to it, "You go not until I set you up a glass / Where you may see . . . / such black and grainèd spots as will not leave their tinct" (*Hamlet* 3.4.20–21, 80–81).[xiii]

Ironism

Richard Rorty has described three conditions for what he calls the ironist perspective:

1. Someone taking this perspective has radical and continuing doubts about the final vocabulary she currently uses, because she has been impressed by other vocabularies, vocabularies taken as final by people or books she has encountered;

2. She realizes that argument phrased in her present vocabulary can neither underwrite nor dissolve these doubts;

---

xii Critique consists "in showing how the existing social order does not allow members, or some of them, fully to realize the potentialities constitutive of their humanity." Boltanski, *On Critique*.

xiii As Foucault said, "The role of the intellectual is no longer to situate himself 'slightly ahead' or 'slightly to one side' so he may speak the silent truth of each and all; it is rather to struggle against those forms of power where he is both instrument and object." G. Deleuze and M. Foucault, "Intellectuals and Power" (1972), in Deleuze, *Desert Islands and Other Texts* (Los Angeles: Semiotext(e), 2004), 207.

3. Insofar as she philosophizes about her situation, she does not
   think that her vocabulary is closer to reality than others, that
   it is in touch with a power not herself.[47]

Anthropologists George Marcus and Michael Fischer add:

> Irony is unsettling: it is a self-conscious mode that senses the failure
> of all sophisticated conceptualizations; stylistically, it employs rhe-
> torical devices that signal real or feigned disbelief on the part of the
> author toward the truth of his own statements; it often centers on
> the recognition of the problematic nature of language, the poten-
> tial foolishness of all linguistic characterizations of reality; and so it
> revels—or wallows—in satirical techniques.[48]

Ironists therefore promote *their* [sic][xiv] ideas through redescriptions, rather than arguments. Accordingly, by combining
critical thinking,[49] *Hua-yen* relationalism,[50] clinical medicine,[51]
and an ironist perspective, this book proceeds by way of a series
of redescriptions.

Q: What is decoloniality?

A: Decoloniality "unsettles the singular authoritativeness and
universal character typically assumed and portrayed in academic
thought. . . . [It] seeks connections and correlations . . . illuminat-
ing pluriversal and interversal paths that disturb the totality from
which the universal and the global are most often perceived. . . .
[It] is necessarily tied to the lived contexts of struggle, struggles
against the structures, matrices, and manifestations of modernity/
coloniality/capitalism/heteropatriarchy, among other structural,
systemic, and systematic modes of power, and for the possibilities of an otherwise. . . . [It] is the process and project of building,

---

xiv Since, as I mentioned previously, ideas can be conceived of as network dialogue rather than belonging to specific individuals.

shaping, and enabling coloniality's otherwise. . . . [It] demands changing the terms of the conversations and making visible the tricks and the designs of the puppeteer: it aims at altering the principles and assumptions of knowledge creation, transforma- tion, and dissemination. . . . [Its] epistemic praxis targets the con- ceptual narratives that sustain and legitimize the implementation of Western global designs."[52]

Redescription (R) Outline

- By way of flash fiction, R1 tells the story of an individual who, after an encounter with Indra's Jewel Net, undergoes an identity change.

- R2 recasts Plato's famous Cave as a Warren to make it more consistent with pluriversal notions of truth (epistemological pluralism or intellectual polycentrism).

- In the tradition of Nacirema ethnography,[53] R3 provides an anthropological account of UN agencies, nongovernmen- tal organizations (NGOs), and research institutes and their involvement in the 2013–2016 Ebola outbreak in West Africa.

- This is followed by a semiotic analysis (R4) of Ebola contain- ment discourse emanating from UN agencies, academia, and rural West Africans in order to analyze the pragmatic ade- quacy of the intellectual categories they employ.[54]

- R5 is a reprint of a short commentary in *The Lancet Global Health* that bears the title "The Ebola Suspect's Dilemma."[55] I interpret this commentary, subsequent letters to the editor, and the authors' reply as a "call and response," which is a discursive practice particularly notable in sub-Saharan Africa where an interlocutor chants an initial phrase and a second group rejoins as a direct commentary on the first. In it, the interlocutors hash out differing views on the symbolic power of public health discourse.

- R6 is an attempt to delink epidemiological knowledge production from the (neo)colonial matrix of power.[56] The first half traces the promises of Big Data for epidemic surveillance and containment, including the manner in which it empirically parses, categorizes, and theoretically explains large swaths of human suffering, concluding that its methodology is mainly a higher-terabyte apparatus for investing neoliberal, bourgeois views of the world with scientific legitimacy.[57] As such, the analysis attempts to explain how mass suffering continues despite enormous economic and technological progress in the Global North, while unveiling the process by which moral norms are tempered. The second half posits epidemiology as an Althusserian ideological apparatus (i.e., as an institution which reproduces the conditions of the social order)[58] through which practitioners use the causal inference paradigm and unwittingly propagate the conditions of global apartheid.

- Based on my research on Ebola vaccine acceptance conducted as part of the NIH's Partnership for Research on Ebola Virus in Liberia PREVAC study (ClinicalTrials.gov: NCT02876328) as well as experience conducting Ebola vaccination campaigns during the 2018–2020 outbreak in the Democratic Republic of the Congo, R7 explores Ebola source theories as a praxis of decoloniality (essentially via a *reductio ad absurdum* of the Habermasian ideal speech situation).

- R8 is an exercise in counterhegemonic computational modeling that explores how HIV preexposure prophylaxis (PrEP) programs give normative dignity to technocratic imperatives while medicalizing gender inequality.[59]

- Prior to the Conclusion, there are Pre-Appendices which contain some R code, the Nkrumahtic Oath, disruptive social media, an analysis of stigma as a form of stigma, and an insurrectional consent form.

- I conclude the book with a call for an Epistemic Reformation and an Afterword anent the COVID-19 pandemic.

Eugene Richardson [@Real_Ironist]

Beni, Democratic Republic of the Congo

June 2019

Redescription 1
Colonizer, Interrupted (Flash Fiction)

The following is not a story about baby shoes for sale, never worn. It is about the half of humanity that cannot afford them.

Flash fiction is a literary mode, usually under 1,000 words, which distills an odyssey. The nanotale about the baby shoes, apocryphally attributed to Hemingway, is one example. The following bildungs*mini*roman—not my personal biography—is another:

Colonizer, Interrupted

We begin with a white upper-middle-class male settler-colonist privilege-exerciser called Quesalid, after the famous shaman of the Pacific Northwest (settler-colonists have no qualms naming people or places after human groups they've decimated). His childhood was typical—summers in Rangoon, luge lessons.

He attended a private boarding school, then some Ivy for college—a common path for mediocre children of rich families attempting to reproduce their elite position in society.[1] It was there that he cemented his masculine identity by participating in the ritual alcohol-poisoning of an acquaintance named Vilmer.

After graduating—diploma in one hand and trust fund in the other—he set out to explore the world. During a two-week stint voluntouring in some godforsaken place his country helped underdevelop,[2] Quesalid became known for his prowess at chucking bags of rice. Around that time, he was transformed by the sight of an aged man, then a sick man, then a corpse, then an ascetic.

At the expat lounge nearby, he decided to take some magic mushrooms to process these *Four Passing Sights*. While tripping, he met a man named Francis, who told him a scintillating tale:

> Far away in the heavenly abode of the great god Indra, there is a wonderful net which has been hung by some cunning artificer in such a manner that it stretches out infinitely in all directions. In accordance with the extravagant tastes of deities, the artificer has hung a single glittering jewel in each "eye" of the net, and since the net itself is infinite in dimensions, the jewels are infinite in number. There hang the jewels glittering like stars of the first magnitude, a wonderful sight to behold. If we now arbitrarily select one of these jewels for inspection and look closely at it, we will discover that in its polished surface there are reflected *all* the other jewels in the net, infinite in number. Not only that, but each of the jewels reflected in this one jewel is also reflecting all the other jewels, so that there is an infinite reflecting process occurring . . .[3]

Quesalid came to the next day in a pineapple field and decided to use his trust fund to scour the world for similar revelations.

In Abya Yala,[i] he discovered *vincularidad*,[4] an "awareness of the integral relation and interdependence amongst all living organisms (in which humans are only a part) with territory or land and the cosmos."[5] In China, he came upon the *Hua-yen*

---

i Abya Yala is an indigenous term used to designate what became known as the Americas (my translation of the Spanish translation of the Tule Kuna). Source: M. López-Hernández, *Encuentros en los senderos de Abya Yala* (Havana: Casa de Las Américas, 2001).

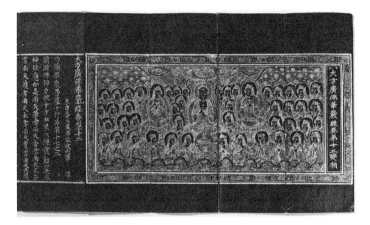

Figure 4
Avataṃsaka Sūtra, vol. 12, frontispiece in gold and silver text on indigo blue paper, mid 14th century.

tradition,[6] which teaches the mutual interfusion and interconnectedness of all phenomena (see figure 4 for further detail). In Africa, he took part in *Ubuntu*, that is, the universal bond that connects all humanity.[7] Last and least in Europe, he experienced *radical relationality*,[8] after which he underwent an identity crisis.

It suddenly dawned on Quesalid that as a white male citizen of the First World, his privilege derived from a racialized, patriarchal, hierarchical, asymmetrical, imperial, heteronormative, neoliberal, and Euro-American-centric order.[9]

"You are a colonizer through and through," he thought. "You can feel it your bones, which have never known stunting. It courses through your veins, through which malaria never has. Every fiber of your being has been nurtured by centuries of predatory accumulation.[10]

"This might serve as a good start to a book," he concluded.

Redescription 2
The Allegory of the Warren (Platonic Dialogues)

In Book VII of Plato's *Republic*, Socrates and Glaucon have a dialogue that presents the famous allegory of the cave. In this scenario, people are chained in a cave and view shadows on a wall that they take for reality. One of their group escapes aboveground and finds Truth in the light of the sun, then returns to disabuse *his*—the truthfinder is specifically masculine—peers of their illusions.

Such a notion of universal truth is at the heart of the coloniality of knowledge, since "the Western/masculinist idea that we can produce knowledges that are unpositioned, unlocated, neutral, and universalistic is one of the most pervasive mythologies in the modern/colonial world."[1]

In *Humanitarian Reason: A Moral History of the Present*, Didier Fassin uses the cave allegory to elucidate the position of the social scientist: s/he is on the threshold of the cave and can slide between there and aboveground so as to render objective critique.[2] Such a heuristic maneuver, however, still suffers from the notion that there is a sun.

To decolonize global health, we must give up such celestial yearnings. That is, we must reject the notion that social inquiry can produce objective, value-neutral, and univocal understanding. Instead, we must embrace the critical and the polyvocal . . . here's how that might look:

The Allegory of the Warren[i]

> Q: Who is Kwame Nkrumah?
>
> A: Kwame Nkrumah was a Ghanaian philosopher and revolution-ary. He was the first prime minister and president of Ghana and is known for his brilliant analyses of neocolonialism and his dedica-tion to pan-Africanism.

[Nkrumah] And now, I said, let me show in a figure how there are multiple vocabularies for representing the world:—Behold! human beings living in an underground warren, which has a Matrix of nests connected by an even greater number of tunnels; here they have been from their childhood, and have their legs and necks chained so that they cannot move, and can only see before them, being prevented by the chains from turning round their heads. Above and behind them are fires blazing at a distance, and between the fires and the prisoners there are raised platforms; and you will see, if you look, low walls built along the platforms, like the screen which marionette players have in front of them, over which they show the puppets.

[Peirce] I see.

---

i Modeled on Plato's *Republic* and the *Zhaungzi* (莊子), a foundational text of Taoism which uses famous historical figures as characters in a dialogue.

> Q: Who is Charles Peirce?
>
> A: Charles Sanders Peirce was an American semiotician who is sometimes considered "the father of pragmatism."

[Nkrumah] And do you see people passing along the wall carrying all sorts of vessels, and statues and figures of animals made of wood and stone and various materials, which appear over the wall?

[Peirce] You have shown me a strange image, and they are strange prisoners.

[Nkrumah] Like ourselves; and they see only the shadows which the fires throw on the opposite walls of the nests?

[Peirce] Indeed.

[Nkrumah] And would you agree these shadows would be the only truth they knew?

[Peirce] But of course. How could they know anything but the shadows if they were never allowed to move their heads?

[Nkrumah] Now look again and see what will naturally follow if the prisoners become aware of this process. At first, when any of them is liberated and compelled suddenly to stand up and turn zir neck round and find that some in the nest weren't chained at all, ze will suffer pains; and those pains will become sharper when ze realizes that those who weren't in chains imposed the set of illusions they came to believe in; that their mental universe had been colonized.[3]

[Peirce] I suppose one of them could then run outside the warren and tell people about the real world aboveground?

[Nkrumah] Nonsense! Nothing exists outside the warren![4] The point of Archimedes is the essence of coloniality.

[Peirce] So whence new vocabularies?[5] New ways of seeing the world?

[Nkrumah] Similar liberations go on in other nests, and without chains our interlocutors are free to roam, tunnel by tunnel, nest to nest.

[Peirce] And why stop at any one in particular?

[Nkrumah] Some are more appealing aesthetically. Some expand the notion of what "we" means. Some have justice as an end. Others . . .

[Peirce] Go on.

[Nkrumah] Others are bigger; they serve to recapture the imagination, to enslave, to co-opt. We call them hegemonic.

[Peirce] Then why not avoid those nests altogether?

[Nkrumah] Ay, there's the rub. There is many a pitfall in the tunnels.

[Peirce] How so?

[Nkrumah] There exists a collection of guides, chaperones, that claim to slide in and out of the warren. And they are programmed by the idea of "the universal" to direct people to the One Nest.

[Peirce] The One that enslaves?

[Nkrumah] The One that enslaves . . . their minds mind you.

[Peirce] So we must rid the warren of these guides.

[Nkrumah] Easier said than done, Charles. They are inveigled by the demands of grants, career aspirations, and the categories of thought supplied by their professional educations.[6]

Q: How do pragmatists view the world?

A: Pragmatism views "social reality as being constantly in flux . . . knowledge as relative and shaped by multiple and instrumentalist goals . . . society as a form of discursive interaction . . . the self as a biographical project free of metaphysical baggage . . . science as will to meaning and power, and . . . methodology as a form of situated inquiry. . . . Contemporary critical pragmatists supplement this view with an emphasis on the construction of reality as a struggle between conflicting discourses and competing definitions of the situation."[7]

[Peirce] Like a form of artificial intelligence: capable of stunning feats of calculation, yet without critical tools to know *what what it does does*.

[Nkrumah] Indeed. They are robbing their wards of a pragmatist notion of truth.[8]

[Peirce] I like where this is going.

[Nkrumah] That every nest has the potential for truth. With the caveat that *truths are illusions about which one has forgotten that this is what they are.*

[Peirce] You mean pluriversalism, as opposed to the failing universalism predicated on Euro-American hegemonic epistemologies?[9] A pluriversalism in which there can exist a truly equal and horizontal communication and dialogue between peoples that goes beyond the logics and practices of domination and exploitation characteristic of the One Nest?[10]

[Nkrumah] And now you understand?

[Peirce] The Truth?

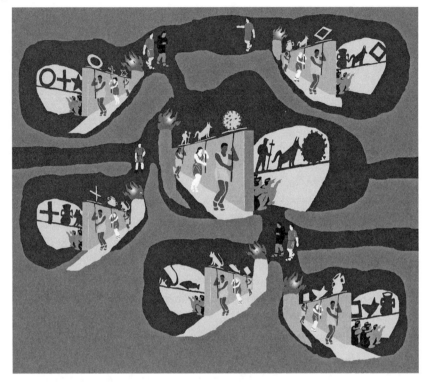

Figure 5
"The Warren," illustration by Lena Gustafson based on a design by
Eugene Richardson.

[**Nkrumah**] Not really, just a more just way of viewing the
world . . . I hope you'll agree.

[**Peirce**] I do . . . Amandla!!

Redescription 3
The Pacification of the Primitive Tribes of Lake Geneva (*Nacirema* Ethnography)[i]

Based on off-the-verandah participant observation and in-depth interviews conducted both in Switzerland and Sierra Leone, the following commissioned report on the international response to the 2013–2016 Ebola outbreak in West Africa (#46 in a distinguished series of After-Action Reports[1] mostly written by authors who performed no action in the field) presents my observations across four thematic areas:

(1) the pacification of a bold social justice agenda in global health by cults of cost-effectiveness and bureaucratic iron cages;

(2) the pacification of a global health ethic by condoning uncivilized research programs lacking clinical delivery platforms;

(3) the pacification of rapid care delivery through the tribal shunning of partnerships;

---

i The *Nacirema* are a group living in North America, whose extensive mouth rites were described by Miner in 1956. Italicized words in this style of ethnography can be read backward for added effect. See H. Miner, "Body Ritual among the Nacirema," *American Anthropologist* 58, no. 3 (1956): 503–507.

(4) the pacification of therapeutic courage by a savage reliance on containment-by-isolation rituals and the magico-religious fetishizing of purpose-built Ebola Treatment Units.

The report ultimately bears witness to the monstrous specter *Ytilainoloc*, who haunts global public health.

The Pacification of the Primitive Tribes of Lake Geneva

> Looking from far and above, from our high places of safety in [African society], it is easy to see all the crudity and irrelevance of [bureaucracy]. But without its power and guidance primitive man could not have mastered his practical difficulties as he has done, nor could man have advanced to the higher stages of civilization.
> —*Ikswonilam Walsinorb* (1948)[2]

I. Executive Summary

The Ebola pandemic[3] that began in 2013 exposed deep inadequacies in the international institutions responsible for protecting the public from the far-reaching biosocial consequences of infectious disease outbreaks.[4] The pandemic raised a critical question: why were the incidence and mortality associated with Ebola virus disease (EVD) so high in West Africa as opposed to the rest of the world?[5] To address this question, Chinua Achebe posthumously commissioned a study of the pacification of the primitive tribes of Lake Geneva,[6] tribes whose peculiar customs and beliefs have long played a leading role in shaping the practices of "global health." Since the magical beliefs and practices of these barbarians have rarely been studied ethnographically, it seemed desirable to investigate them as an example of the extremes to which human behavior can go.

II. The Iron Cage of Global Health

After visiting European archives, I discovered parchments scribed over a century ago by *Rebew*, an *inyanga* (isiZulu: diviner) from the Chiefdom of Saxony. In oracular fashion, he predicted that, as societies became more efficient and rationally organized under the spirit of capitalism, humans would begin to find themselves trapped in a system based purely on technological efficiency and instrumental action. He labeled this trap the "iron cage," and called its predominant inhabitants *Tarcuaerub*.

This divination has found its apotheosis in the *OHW*, a tribe of *Tarcuaerub* and medicine-persons, dedicated to providing technical advice to improve the health of people they rarely—if ever—meet (essentially a form of dumb barter[ii] where the *Tarcuaerub* receive numerous CSEs [cowry shell equivalents] for their advice). After three stints as a participant observer at the *OHW* Takienta[iii] (figure 6) in Geneva, I was able establish sufficient rapport to examine their relics and join their rituals.

OHW culture is predominantly characterized by an activity they call *gnihsup-repap*. They also spend many hours each day in front of luminous tablets, through which they communicate with each other. Via a silicon-based Kula Ring,[7] the *Tarcuaerub* circulate ephemeral objects they call *liam-e*. *Liam-e* are rarely held onto for long, but rather forwarded through a complex network where the mere act of such circulation substitutes for

---

ii Dumb barter is a kind of exchange system in which the parties avoiding personal contact leave goods at accepted locations in return for other items. G. O. Faure, "Dumb Barter: A Seminal Form of Negotiation," *Negotiation Journal* 27, no. 4 (2011): 403–418.

iii Takienta is the Ditammari word for tower-house. The Tammari are significantly more developed than the *Tarcuaerub* and reside in West Africa.

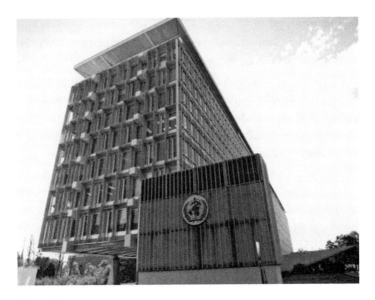

Figure 6
OHW Takienta.

field labor. Indeed, the *OHW* was heavily criticized for not taking decisive field action at the time it confirmed the circulation
of Ebola virus in West Africa in March 2014.[8] As one informant
put it, "When thousands of people start bleeding out of their
mouths and eyes, sometimes it's best to take a step back and see
where it's all going."[9]

The *OHW* tribe and their social science mercenaries also
played a role in promoting culturalist claims of causality[10]
regarding the genesis of the Ebola outbreak.[11] Together, they
have taken a blood oath with an anti-politics witch[12] to convert
all political-economic phenomena into technical bits amenable
to spirit mediation by social scientists and medicine-persons.
Thus, I heard their tribespersons chant, for example: "traditional

burial practices played a major role in the spread of Ebola virus." It would be taboo to say, "transnational relations of inequality played a major role in its spread,"[13] as the tribe would lose a great deal of cowry shell equivalents from their Paramount Chiefs.

One of the most vociferous *OHW* House Societies[14] is a cult dedicated to the deity *Ssenevitceffe Tsoc*. Belief in this deity causes cult followers to measure the value of human life in cowry shell equivalents. More often than not, the darker the complexion of the human, the fewer CSEs allotted. Over the years, this cult has opposed the treatment of multidrug-resistant tuberculosis in Peru, because the expense was too great for the tribespersons to bear.[15] Similar arguments were made against introducing antiretroviral therapy to Africans with HIV/AIDS.[16] Despite this fealty to *Ssenevitceffe Tsoc*, both arguments were successfully combatted by scholactivist clans.[17]

Unfortunately, the inertia of these treatment taboos carries over to other diseases. As will be discussed in the next section, the *Tarcuaerub*'s primeval fear of diverting money from preventive measures paradoxically results in the preventable deaths of an untold number of non-*Tarcuaerub* (who are considered second-class organisms).[18]

III. The Containment Mystique

Since the colonial period in West Africa, the dominant logic for epidemic disease containment (including smallpox, malaria, and influenza) has dictated isolation of sick individuals, with little in the way of patient care.[19] Thus, it was not surprising in my clinical work in 2014–2015 to find that many Ebola temples simply functioned to isolate sick patients while at most providing oral rehydration, even to those with severe vomiting. (People dying of hypovolemic shock—that is, the condition where there is not enough fluid in the circulatory system to perfuse the major organs—need fluid replacement. If they cannot take it orally on account of vomiting, then the best way to provide it is intravenously [IV]. You can imagine, then, the pain-frustration of holding cups of ORS[iv] to dying Ebola patients' mouths and seeing them vomit it back up, knowing full well the IVs we desperately wanted to use were 100 feet away in the green zone . . . but their use was banned by the Paramount Chiefs in Belgium [more on this below in "Tribal Fetishes"].)

Despite ritual wailing by the *FSM* tribe, the international containment response did not begin in earnest until the *OHW* tribe sounded a magic chant eight months after the first documented case: "Public Health Emergency of International Concern . . . Public Health Emergency of International Concern . . . Public Health Emergency of International Concern."[20] As an extension of the isolation-over-treatment fetish, one could posit high-income-country biosecurity as the primary rationalization for tardy "aid" delivery.[21] This "foraging" for biosecurity supports the claim that Guinea, Sierra Leone, and Liberia were used by the hordes of the Global North as a large West Africa Ebola Holding Unit[22] (rather than view each of the Ebola isolation facilities set up in the three countries as separate holding units, a counter-hegemonic use of the phrase might view the entire region as a single holding unit for the Global North [given the fact that high-income-country biosecurity—not the provision of high-level care for EVD—was the primary logic for international contributions to containment]).

---

iv Oral rehydration salts—essentially Gatorade for dehydrated patients.

IV. Savage Rituals

Some of the most savage rituals I witnessed in these attempts to contain the Ebola pandemic were the research-without-clinical-delivery rites. Akin to cannibalism, these rites sacrifice human lives to certain deities, in this case a particularly monstrous cosmic being named *Latipac Cimedaca*, who has been studied by the sociologist Pierre Bourdieu.[23] While under the trance of *Latipac Cimedaca*, cult members are incited to extract valuable, career-advancing "data" directly from the bodies of ill individuals—but are not compelled to provide any medical assistance in return.

These rites were notably performed in the Kenema district of Sierra Leone, where tens of millions of US dollars were used by a university consortium for biodefense research, with very little earmarked for clinical care. We thus witnessed the most absurd and tragic of phenomena: that of a shiny, well-resourced research laboratory next to a dilapidated, resource-poor hospital[v] (@real_DrPH[vi]).[24] Despite the heroic efforts of *OHW* and Sierra Leonean medicine-persons, many of the latter, and many of their patients, perished because of the lack of prioritization of clinical care.[25]

Research-without-clinical-delivery rites also engender witchcraft. For example, the aforementioned research group lacked a clinical delivery platform to treat Ebola patients; however, it had invented a rapid-diagnostic test for Ebola for which it needed patient samples to validate its effectiveness. They therefore sent a Research-Assistant-Witch (or RAW) to use his stealthy powers to

---

v It reminded me of my time at Duke University, where a "Gothic wonderland" with an $8 billion endowment stood next to the dilapidated, resource-poor town of Durham, North Carolina.

vi A DrPH is also the doctoral degree offered by schools of public health.

surreptitiously enter other groups' Ebola temples to draw unauthorized blood samples. He was eventually exorcised, and the study was transferred to a group whose RAs lacked such sorcery. As Van De Grijspaarde (2013) notes, witchcraft often manifests in areas of normative—and in this case, ethical—ambiguity.[26]

V. Tribal Fetishes

The tribes of Lake Geneva are obsessed with a deity they call *Ytefasrekrowerachtlaeh*, to the extent that they are blinded toward alliances with other tribes. For example, our Liberian and Sierra Leonean informants who worked for their respective health ministries told us that one fiercely independent tribe in particular, *FSM*, was notoriously difficult to partner with in terms of shared agendas. Their subservience to the *Ytefasrekrowerachtleah* deity led to justifications of therapeutic nihilism, where clinicians at Ebola temples were barred from placing IVs in EVD patients dying from shock, because it was deemed to be too dangerous or relatively ineffectual[27] by their Paramount Chiefs in Belgium.[28]

By contrast, another tribe, *Htlaeh Ni Srentrap (HIP)*, worshiped a competing deity called *Secivresfotnemyolpeddipar*. *HIP*, a warrior caste known for its effectiveness in health systems strengthening, migrated to Sierra Leone in October 2014 and was requested by the president of that country to focus its activity in Port Loko, due to a surge in cases and lack of any functional international presence in that district. Several other tribes responded to similar entreaties, and the district Ebola response got under way. Within two weeks, *HIP* was operating an Ebola temple converted from a vocational training center, in cooperation with the Ministry of Health. The set-up was not ideal for infection prevention and control, but the twin mandates of prioritizing patient care and

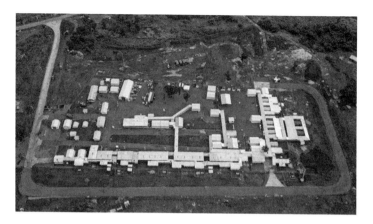

Figure 7
Ebola temple.

government involvement impelled *HIP* to begin work under conditions where other tribes would not.

For these other tribes, the aforementioned *Ytefasrekrow-erachtleah* was the deity of choice: they thus constructed self-contained Ebola temples that took months to complete (figure 7), during which time the health ministry and *HIP* bore the brunt of the Port Loko response.

But did *HIP*'s focus on patients result in unsafe conditions for its tribespersons? Despite award-winning infotainment that advances such a presumption,[29] the evidence suggests otherwise. The Ebola temples operated by *FSM* in West Africa treated 4,962 confirmed cases during which time 14 of their health care workers died from EVD.[30] The facilities operated by *HIP* treated 630 confirmed cases, during which time 1 health care worker died. Thus, *FSM* had 1 staff fatality per 354 patients treated; by comparison, *HIP* had 1 staff fatality per 630 patients treated.

HIP also demonstrated a significantly improved case fatality rate (CFR): 49% (179/366) vs. 58% (187/324); Chi-square p = 0.009,[vii] after controlling for survival bias[31] (i.e., comparing CFRs from patients who traveled less than 100 km to the Ebola unit in question, since the sickest patients often die before being transferred from far-off holding centers). This was likely on account of *HIP*'s more aggressive (i.e., warrior-caste)[viii] treatment approach.[32]

One could thus conclude that self-contained Ebola temples that eschew government involvement do not necessarily result in safer conditions for staff, nor do they equate with better treatment outcomes.

VI. Conclusion

A specter is haunting global health—the specter of *Ytilainoloc*.
—*Tsohg S'xram Lrak* (2020)

Contrary to numerous After-Action Report claims, the 2013-2016 Ebola outbreak in West Africa should not be seen as a failure of the international system.[33] Foraging on the periphery's resources by core countries of the Global North—also known as predatory accumulation[34]—and concomitant subaltern underdevelopment[35] constitute the world system as it was constructed to work.[36] Indeed, the *OHW* and other *NU* institutions are meant

---

vii The *FSM* tribe had an overall CFR of 51% (260/505) reported in those for whom an address was available (96% of cases). The CFR for those who traveled more than 100 km to the ETU was 40% (73/181), and these were removed from the above analysis as a correction for survival bias.

viii Warrior castes are known for monitoring vital signs, putting in IVs and intraosseous needles, and checking electrolyte levels and renal function.

to be toothless interventionists. Only when global bi(
was threatened did they become drivers of "aid." Morec
the dominant containment-only logic prevailed across numerous tribes shows that the coloniality of global health praxis has
yet to be dismantled.

Research enterprises lacking clinical delivery platforms
should be seen as part of this coloniality. It results in scenarios
where foreign universities (Krio: strangers) extract academic capital without providing a commensurable offering to health care
shrines. Indeed, I see this as the preeminent bioethical concern
of contemporary global health.

One final conclusion concerns the duration of tribal migration in response to epidemics. The very notion of a bounded
"outbreak" is problematic as it obscures the transnational and
translocal historical forces that coalesce over time to manifest
as human pathology.[37] When tribes left the region once West
Africa reached "zero Ebola," I was left wondering: Can the traveling circus of humanitarian relief and epidemic research deliver
sustained improvements in global health?

Redescription 4
WHO's Semiosis (Semiotics)

Semiotics helps us to not take representations for granted as reflections of reality, enabling us to take them apart and consider whose realities they represent.

—Daniel Chandler, *Semiotics: The Basics* (2002)

The structural and material determinants of infectious disease epidemics have been well described, and an epistemic community has formed around understanding the processes by which social forces become embodied as pathology.[1] Less attention has been paid, however, to examining the ideological content of how diseases are represented.[2] In the following redescription, I suggest ways to explore the semiotics of outbreak containment, including how we might interrogate the models, graphs, and terminology deployed by UN agencies and academic epidemiologists. How do these apparently neutral descriptors construct a worldview that reproduces coloniality? In other words, how do these Have-istemic communities ultimately commit symbolic violence?

WHO's Semiosis

> Whenever a sign is present, ideology is present too.
> —Валентин Николаевич Волошинов, *Marxism and the Philosophy of Language* (1929)

I. NEJM-Editor 1:18–25

The 2013–2016 Ebola pandemic[3] was the longest and largest on record.[4] Since its conception was traced, in rather immaculate epidemiological fashion, to a two-year-old Guinean in December 2013 anno Domini,[5] there has been no shortage of strategy papers, reviews, viewpoints, commentaries, projections, lessons learned, and After-Action Reports published (R3, for example). While such accounts have "exposed deep inadequacies in the national and international institutions responsible for protecting the public" and recommended reforms accordingly,[6] they also uncritically impart epistemological currency to certain neocolonial vocabularies so as to invest them with scientific legitimacy.[7]

To gain insight into this distorting process, one can employ discourse analysis and pragmatic semiotics (i.e., the study of how reality is represented—and indeed constructed—through signs, including words, figures, graphs, models, etc.).[8] In the redescription that follows, I review Ebola containment discourse emanating from UN agencies, academia, and rural West Africans in order to analyze the pragmatic adequacy of the intellectual categories they employ.[9] Where such categories reflect an affirmation of the status quo—essentially that of certain powerful interests—I critique them as unjust.[10] Where they reflect otherwise, they may be used as grist for the mill of decoloniality.

II. UN Agencies

The World Health Organization (WHO) was widely criticized for its initial response to the Ebola outbreak in West Africa, even receiving calls for its dissolution and the creation of a new global health agency.[11] My present aim is not to further critique the UN agency's failure to provide decisive leadership despite clear evidence the epidemic was out of control.[12] Rather, I mean to draw attention to the more subtle, discursive means by which the WHO paradoxically exacerbates and naturalizes the very inequalities it aspires to redress.[13]

Despite its mission "to ensure the highest attainable level of health for all people,"[14] the WHO is no stranger to amplifying epidemics. In the 1990s, their intransigent stance on treating all cases of tuberculosis (TB) with first-line antibiotic regimens led to an increased incidence of multidrug resistance in countries such as Russia and Peru.[15] Subsequently Paul Farmer showed how the production, content, and dispersal of "scientific knowledge" about such TB epidemics were molded by a series of hegemonic (and thus often unexamined) ideologies tightly tied to neoliberal economics. Such ideology, he wrote, shaped "not only the dissemination of knowledge—through the promotion of officially condoned treatment strategies for tuberculosis—but also the very construction of our categories of evidence."[16]

And while the WHO often ultimately rectifies its official condoning of inequitable treatment strategies (e.g., endorsing DOTS-Plus as a response to the first half of Farmer's critique),[17] it rarely examines—let alone amends—its discursive practices (the second half of his critique).[i]

---

i The four stages of WHO acceptance of evidence related to global health equity:

1. This is worthless nonsense.
2. This is an interesting, but perverse, point of view.
3. This is true, but quite unimportant.
4. We always said so.

Source: J. B. S. Haldane, "Review of The Truth about Death," Journal of Genetics 58 (1963): 464.

For example, in a report entitled "After Ebola in West Africa—Unpredictable Risks, Preventable Epidemics," the WHO Ebola Response Team devoted a figure to depicting the contribution of "superspreaders" to the outbreak in West Africa (figure 8). They found that approximately 20% of individuals generate 80% of cases of Ebola virus disease (or they just recycled the Pareto principle).[18] Their citation of a 1997 paper by Woolhouse and colleagues implies support for control programs targeted at this "core" 20%.[19]

What looks at first like a benign set of graphs put together by public health experts takes on a different hue when we subject it to Foucault's assertion that "People know what they do, frequently they know why they do what they do, but what they don't know is what what they do does":[20]

(1) *People know what they do.* The coauthors of this article are public health experts.

———————————————————————————————➤

Figure 8

Superspreading of Ebola virus disease according to numbers of infections and geographic distance. In Panel A, the overdispersed distribution of 287 confirmed secondary cases of Ebola virus disease (EVD) arising from primary cases in Conakry, Guinea, is shown at left, with 0 to 8 secondary cases arising from each primary case. Approximately 20% of the primary, confirmed cases generated 80% of the secondary cases, as shown at right. Panel B shows the spread of infection during 2015 in a first generation of confirmed cases in Aberdeen, a coastal neighborhood in Freetown (top graph). One man with EVD fled Aberdeen for the village of Rosanda in the Bombali district, 200 km from the source of the original outbreak, thereby establishing a second, third, and possibly a fourth generation of cases in that village (bottom graph). Source: WHO Ebola Response Team, "After Ebola in West Africa—Unpredictable Risks, Preventable Epidemics," *New England Journal of Medicine* 375, no. 6 (2016): 587–596.

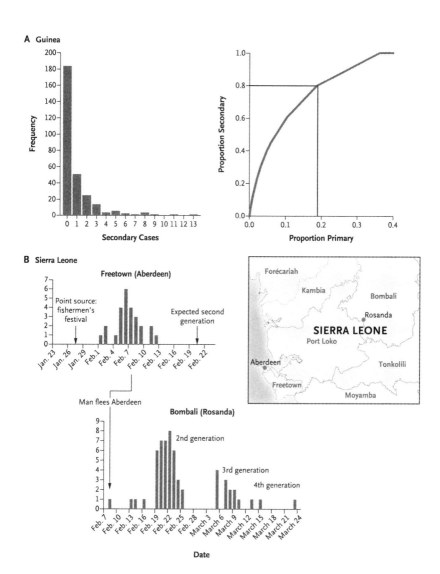

A Guinea

Frequency vs *Secondary Cases*

Proportion Secondary vs *Proportion Primary*

B Sierra Leone

Freetown (Aberdeen)

Point source: fishermen's festival

Expected second generation

Man flees Aberdeen

Bombali (Rosanda)

2nd generation

3rd generation

4th generation

Date

(2) *Frequently they know why they do what they do.* The coauthors are dedicated to improving the health of populations.

(3) *But what they don't know is what what they do does.* They do not realize how they impart epistemological currency to a term like superspreader, which "perniciously diverts us from structural determinants of Ebola virus transmission by positing bounded individuals and their unconstrained, calculating agency . . . as the engines of transmission."[21] As such, tangible sources of exploitation disappear behind the facades of objective rationality.[22]

Q: What is epistemological currency?

A: Epistemological currency can be thought of as the philosophical mechanisms which raise a concept from opinion or interpretation to "true" knowledge or scientific fact.

One will never find a WHO article describing corrupt mining companies as superspreaders,[23] since, in an alienated social formation such as ours,[24] conventional epidemiologists would likely deem such an analysis "political." For the most part, epidemiology as a method of science is considered apolitical; it actually serves as an ideological apparatus of imperialism by shielding the structural causes of health inequities in the Global South.

Furthermore, as part of containment-by-isolation practices that can be traced back to colonial medical schemes in Africa,[25] UN agency publications one year into the outbreak failed to highlight the 0% case fatality rate (CFR) in repatriated American citizens (9/9 survived with the intensive supportive care available at most high-income-country hospitals).[26] This datum should have prompted agency-wide commitments to promote aggressive resuscitation at Ebola treatment [sic][ii] units.[27] Instead, the UN Mission for Ebola Emergency Response (UNMEER) and WHO repeatedly endorsed control measures consisting of patient isolation, safe burial practices, contact tracing, and infection control.[28] Médecins Sans Frontières was one of the few organizations to realize that this bias against treatment was "an institutionalized form of non-assistance" that resulted in "a high number of presumably avoidable deaths."[29] As deduced below in section IV, the high mortality rates that resulted from this lack of prioritization of aggressive treatment likely had the added impact of hampering isolation efforts.

III. Academia

Whatever the poverty, never will it breed disease.
—Louis Pasteur (1888)[30]

Where is the terminology used by UN agencies forged? Much of the technical jargon employed to describe infectious disease outbreaks comes from the discipline of epidemiology, which the WHO defines as "the study of the distribution and determinants of health-related states or events (including disease), and the application of this study to the control of diseases and other health problems."[31]

The discipline has been criticized by the preeminent statistician David Freedman for "using statistical models to avoid the

---

ii [sic] because many of them provided little in the way of treatment (as discussed in R3).

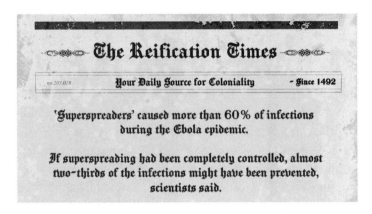

Figure 9
Media ramifications. P. Dockrill, "'Superspreaders' Caused More Than 60% of Infections During the Ebola Epidemic," *ScienceAlert*, 2017; L. H. Sun, "Disease 'Superspreaders' Accounted for Nearly Two-thirds of Ebola Cases, Study Finds," *Washington Post*, 2017.

hard work of examining problems in their full specificity and complexity."[32] Using Ebola transmission models as an example, the following two sections illustrate this critique, showing how armchair exercises carried out on a computer depoliticize complex, historical phenomena into numeric bits amenable to mathematical manipulation, policy recommendations, and technical intervention.[33]

The quotes in figure 9 represent the media ramifications of a 2017 modeling study published by Princeton investigators in the *Proceedings of the National Academy of Sciences* (*PNAS*). The study found[iii] that "superspreaders" played a key role in sustaining

---

iii The authors actually describe "finding that superspreading occurred," which evinces more of a positivist than social-constructivist epistemology.

onward transmission of the Ebola epidemic in West Africa, and these individuals were *responsible* for a significant proportion of infections.[34]

Q: What is the *Maafa*?

A: *Maafa* is the Swahili word for "disaster" or "great tragedy" and is used "to describe the history and ongoing effects of atrocities inflicted on African people, particularly when committed by non-Africans . . . specifically in the context of the history of slavery . . . and argued as 'continued to the present day' through imperialism, colonialism, and other forms of oppression." (https://en.wikipedia.org/wiki/Maafa)

It can be useful to think of *PNAS* and other high-impact journals as validating the types of discourse that society accepts and makes function as true[35]—or, as instruments for enforcing meanings.[36] As deconstructionist philosopher Jacques Derrida points out, violence is implicit in the assignation of meaning.[37] Like the WHO Ebola Response Team's article cited above, Lau and colleagues reify and therefore authenticate the use of "superspreader" as a synchronic epidemiological descriptor of bounded individuals as agents of disease transmission—without lending analytical weight to how sociohistorical forces become embodied as Ebola virus disease. As such, the authors unintentionally (since they are no doubt compassionate global health advocates) function as "transfer mechanisms"[38] for the ideology of predatory accumulation, in essence diverting the public's gaze from legacies of the *Maafa* (or African Holocaust), colonialism, white supremacy, indirect rule, structural adjustment, institutional racism, and extractive foreign companies (I posit this set of candidates as vying for the appelation of "superspreader").[39] *Pace* Lau and colleagues (who notably lack West African coauthors),[40] one can read "residual imperialist propensities"[41] in statements such as: "Understanding superspreading can facilitate devising individually targeted control measures, which may outperform population-level measures"[42]—which could be roughly interpreted as meaning, earmark $3 billion to stop human superspreaders, not corporate ones.

> Q: What do synchronic and diachronic mean?
>
> A: Synchronic inquiry evaluates a phenomenon at a specific point in time, usually the present. Diachronic inquiry considers the genealogy of phenomena over time.

Quaeritur: Does the milder term "superspreading event"[43] obviate the above critiques?

It does not. The removal of individual agency does not compensate for the continued lack of historical scrutiny the term offers. It may be more useful to view the signing of agreements between mining corporations and the governments of Guinea, Sierra Leone, and Liberia—contracts which have resulted in billions of dollars for transnationals yet very little in the way of social benefits, including health infrastructure, for rural populations (due to illicit financial flows)[44]—as superspreading events.[45]

*   *   *

As another example, in a highly cited article in *Science*, Pandey and colleagues develop a stochastic model of Ebola transmission and find "that a combined approach of case isolation, contact-tracing with quarantine, and sanitary funeral practices must be implemented with utmost urgency in order to reverse the growth of the outbreak." They go on to say that "Given the current lack of licensed therapeutic treatments and vaccines, near-term measures to curb transmission must rely on nonpharmaceutical interventions, including quarantine, case isolation, contact precautions, and sanitary burial practices that consist of disinfecting the cadaver before inclosure in a body bag that is further disinfected."[46] The failure to recognize that effective treatment did indeed exist may come as no surprise when it is noted that none of the authors are clinicians. Indeed, if one traces the genealogy of the mathematical models they use, one finds they were developed in the 1920s by a physician (who had joined Ronald Ross on a Sierra Leone malaria campaign that was predicated on prevention despite the existence of quinine)[iv] and a chemist (whose research on the nonagentive action of molecules shines through in the deterministic epidemic models he helped develop).[47] To be fair, I would argue that these omissions regarding treatment occur not by choice but rather by the habit of forcing nature into the conceptual boxes supplied by public health education.[48] Nonetheless, it is clear that the categories supplied by such training—the *déformation professionelle*[49]—have life-and-death consequences.

We thus begin to see a potential category-source for UN agencies' focus on containment over care. Again, the 0% CFR in repatriated American citizens should remind us that EVD is

---

iv It was further based on segregation of Africans and colonizers: one can thus see seeds of racism in the genealogy of epidemic models.

an eminently treatable disease;[v] outbreak containment strategies which neglect this crucial element scuttle an equity agenda[50] and, in so doing, "autoclav[e] imperialism's back story."[51] Another way to approach this is to think of public health science as a mode of artificial intelligence, capable of stunning feats of calculation, yet without critical tools to know *what what it does does*.

IV. Rural West Africans

> There's really no such thing as the "voiceless." There are only the deliberately silenced, or the preferably unheard.
>
> —Arundhati Roy, Sydney Peace Prize Lecture (2004)

My interviews with EVD patients, survivors, and their family members—both as a clinician during the outbreak and as an anthropologist conducting research in its aftermath—provide a different way of understanding the vocabulary employed by epidemiologists to describe Ebola virus transmission in West Africa.[52]

For example, when I discussed the concept of "superspreader" with a number of people affected by the outbreak, not one agreed that using the term to describe individuals was appropriate. Some felt their national governments should be deemed superspreaders because of endemic corruption;[53] others felt foreign corporations were to blame: "Firestone was the superspreader, since their lobbying prevented us from

---

v This occurred before a clinical trial in the DRC demonstrated the effectiveness of monoclonal antibody treatments. S. Mulangu, L. E. Dodd, R. T. Davey, et al., "A Randomized, Controlled Trial of Ebola Virus Disease Therapeutics," *New England Journal of Medicine* 381 (2019): 2293–2303.

getting a tire factory"; a few discussed the legacy of the African Holocaust.[54]

In addition, when contacts of survivors who were sick during active Ebola transmission in their village were asked why they avoided presenting to an Ebola treatment [sic] unit, most described fear, stigma,[vi] that "no one came out alive," and distrust of government and international institutions as reasons. However, when I proposed the hypothetical scenario in which two out of every three patients survived admission and were discharged—not at all implausible at an ETU which provided aggressive intravenous resuscitation—most indicated they would have attended. This raises the question whether containment efforts in West Africa were indeed hampered by a focus on isolation only.

V. Colonial Amplification

Figure 10 shows a sign that was posted throughout Sierra Leone recommending that individuals with signs and symptoms consistent with Ebola virus disease go immediately to their nearest health facility; however, once epidemiologists realized that health facilities were *amplifying* Ebola virus transmission, they instead advised that people stay home, remain isolated, and call the emergency number 117 to receive help.

---

vi Using "stigma" in this conventional fashion, that is, as a term to connote discrimination against people infected (or thought to be) with Ebola virus, HIV, or some other pathogen, bewitches our intelligence into overlooking the stigma that causes higher risk for these infections in the first place: namely, the global "racial theater" that is the space of systematic stigmatization (see Pre-Appendix 四). Source: A. Mbembe, *Critique of Black Reason* (Durham: Duke University Press, 2017).

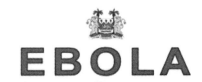

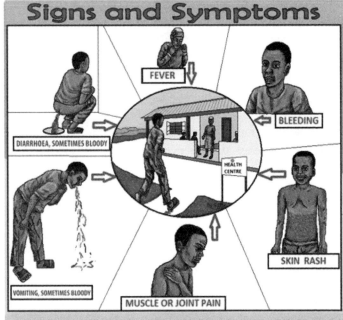

Figure 10
UNICEF poster.

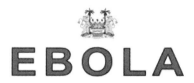

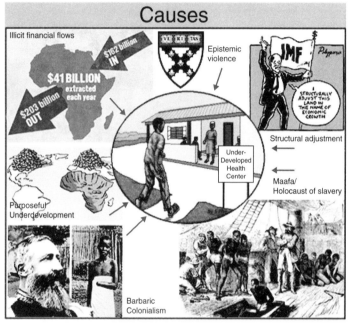

Figure 11
Decoloniality poster.

As a reminder that seemingly neutral public health messages are not impervious to recontextualization[55] (and as an exercise in decoloniality), figure 11 modifies this sign to show how purposefully underdeveloped health infrastructures *amplify* transnational inequities.

Redescription 5
The Ebola Suspect's Dilemma (Call and Response)

Group 1: "Amandla! (Power!)"
Group 2: "Awethu! (To us!)"
—South African rallying cry

"Call and response" is a discursive practice that stems from a variety of traditions but is particularly notable in sub-Saharan Africa. After an interlocutor chants an initial phrase, a second group rejoins as a direct commentary on the first.

> Q: What is symbolic violence?
>
> A: Symbolic violence can be thought of as "the capacity to impose the means for comprehending and adapting to the social world by representing the economic and political world in disguised, taken-for-granted forms."[1]

The Ebola Suspect's Dilemma

Our ideas on the *origin* of epidemiological prejudices received provisional expression in a brief commentary in *The Lancet Global Health* that bears the title "The Ebola Suspect's Dilemma."[2] This commentary, subsequent letters to the editor, and authors' reply can be viewed as a "call and response"—one between coauthors and "collaborating" respondents.[3] In it, *we* demonstrate differing appreciations for the potential of public health discourse to cause symbolic violence.

The initial call is based on the Israeli economist Ariel Rubinstein's contention that

(1) game theory has little real-world practical utility;

(2) mathematical models are merely fables dressed in formal language (that therefore create the illusion of being scientific);

(3) economics is an academic discipline which tends toward conservativism and helps the privileged in society maintain their dominance.[4]

Public health "science" borrows these fabulistic tools to parse health phenomena, and in so doing imposes conservative, scientistic means for comprehending such phenomena by occulting oppressive power structures.[5] This helps the privileged maintain their dominance by convincing those suffering from Ebola, for example, that they have been harmed by a virus and not by 400 years of predatory accumulation.

The Ebola suspect's dilemma

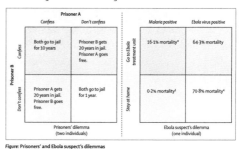

In 1950, Merrill Flood and Melvin Dresher of the RAND Corporation developed a theoretical model of cooperation and conflict, which was later formalised by Albert W Tucker as the prisoner's dilemma.[1] This model represents a situation in which two prisoners each have the option to confess or not, but their sentencing outcomes depend crucially on the simultaneous choice of the other (figure).[1] Fittingly, it has become the paradigmatic example of individual versus group rationality and is an often used heuristic when conveying introductory social theory to students.

Although not a homologous predicament, the Ebola virus disease suspect also faces a consequential dilemma (figure). The 'rational'—that is, not informed by superstition or baseless rumour—aversion to West Africa's ill-equipped and poorly sanitised hospitals was described even before the 2014-16 Ebola outbreak.[2] This characterisation could a fortiori be extended to those Ebola virus disease suspects who eschewed presentation at an Ebola treatment unit, especially those units that offered little in the way of aggressive intravenous resuscitation or management of electrolyte disturbances. Consider the situation in which you are an Ebola virus disease suspect (you have fever, vomiting, muscle pain, and headache), but don't know whether you have Ebola virus disease: (1) if you have undiagnosed malaria and stay at home, your chance of dying is 0·2%;[3] (2) if you have undiagnosed malaria and go to an Ebola treatment unit, your chance of dying from Ebola virus disease is 16·1% (around 25% chance of nosocomial Ebola virus transmission with 64·3% mortality);[4] or (3) if you have Ebola virus disease, stay at home, and self-isolate, your chance of dying is 70·8%.[4] Given equal chances of having malaria (West Africa is the region with the world's highest incidence of malaria) or Ebola virus disease, your overall mortality risk for staying at home is 35·5% versus 40·2% for going to a Ebola treatment unit.

Thus, you would be acting in your rational self-interest by staying at home, since the suspect who is uninfected might become so nosocomially through ambulance transport with actual cases or unsafe triage at an Ebola treatment unit—not factoring in (1) rational desires to die at home rather than in (or in the queue in front of) a far off tent; (2) rational fears that you might never see

your family again; (3) rational responses to the pervasive messaging that Ebola has no cure; or (4) the irony that, once admitted to an Ebola treatment unit that does not offer intravenous volume replacement, a rational decision might be to deliberately infect yourself with malaria: emerging evidence suggests that *Plasmodium* parasitemia offers a greater survival benefit than the oral rehydration approach used at many Ebola treatment units in 2014.[5] And therein lies the Ebola suspect's dilemma—at least according to the rational choice lens that refracts the world around us into binary options for our moral retinas.

Now consider a Special Report[6] by the WHO Ebola Response Team. In it, the authors rightly—if not tautologically—suggest that shortening the delay to isolation of Ebola virus disease suspects would lead to quicker overall outbreak containment, yet they fail to adequately discuss the reality that suspects will continue to be "unwilling to seek medical care,"[6] when such care is non-existent. Indeed, our extensive interviews with survivors of Ebola virus disease and their families reveal—among a variety of reasons for Ebola treatment unit avoidance early in the outbreak—the common suggestion that international non-governmental organisations in future epidemics not be allowed to set up Ebola treatment units if they do not provide intravenous resuscitation as standard of care.

Conversely, if Ebola suspects maximise their chances of survival (by staying at home in the case above), they risk—according to the methodological individualist

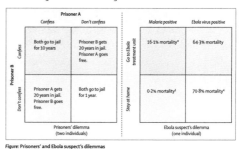

Figure: Prisoners' and Ebola suspect's dilemmas
*Around 25% chance of nosocomial Ebola virus transmission with 64·3% mortality.

framing of a multitude of after action reports—being dubbed "superspreaders"[6] (or rather "vectors"[7] if they actively flee admission to an Ebola treatment unit). Such terminology perniciously diverts us from structural determinants of Ebola virus transmission by positing bounded individuals and their unconstrained, calculating agency—or its contralateral blinder, fear-related behaviour[7] (a term originally applied to lab rats)—as the engines of transmission, and potentially engenders stigmatisation towards patients with Ebola virus disease, including posthumously. We find the descriptor, personal protective equipment (PPE)-bereft care-nexus, more appropriate, both anthropologically and philosophically. It highlights the fact that Ebola virus disease is a caregivers' disease that thrives in underdeveloped[8] and historically plundered regions, and that the use of terms such as superspreader or vector factitiously implicates marginalised individuals as sources of outbreaks, instead of lending analytical weight to how social forces (ie, the complex fields of power in which we are all nodes) become embodied as pathology.[9]

In the final analysis, however, the implication that there is a decision to be made (seek medical care or not) or a 'spreader' to be found is merely a cognitive convention that has been imposed on the PPE-bereft care-nexus by western philosophy. Such language is couched in rational choice models and other scientistic paradigms—that is, technocratic ways of thinking which elevate the formal rationality practised in modern science to a quasi-divine faculty for isolating truth, without considering the plurality of roles that reason can take[10]—which comprise the modern missionary's (ie, aid worker's) faith and sanctify the individual at a specific point in time as opposed to webs of relations and how they change diachronically. These platonic shadows-on-the-wall, so to speak, also divert attention from outside the cave, where legacies of the transatlantic slave trade, colonialism, indirect rule, structural adjustment, and extractive foreign companies—the real superspreaders—have been, and continue to be, embodied as viral disease in West Africa, resulting in the preventable demise of large swaths of humanity.[11]

Therefore, we can view the Ebola suspect's dilemma as a heuristic for the most recent outbreak in West Africa. First, we must temper the fetishisation of containment-through-isolation by a greater commitment to carry out aggressive resuscitation in future infectious disease outbreaks where shock is a predominant feature (evidence for the "injection of saline solutions in extraordinary quantities"[12] in such a scenario existed as early as 1832, but was poorly translated to the 2013–16 outbreak in West Africa). Second, we must recognise the practical and interpretive limits of rationalist epistemologies—including the categories of thought that are instilled by our training as scientists, clinicians, and public health professionals[13]—while exploring paradigms informed by biosocial analysis and methodological relationalism.[14]

*Eugene T Richardson, Mohamed Bailor Barrie, Cameron T Nutt, J Daniel Kelly, Raphael Frankfurter, Mosoka P Fallah, Paul E Farmer
Division of Global Health Equity, Brigham and Women's Hospital, Boston, MA 02115, USA (ETR, PEF); Partners In Health, Freetown, Sierra Leone (ETR, MBB, CTN, JDK, RF, PEF); Department of Anthropology, Stanford University, Stanford, CA, USA (ETR); Department of Global Health and Social Medicine, Harvard Medical School, Boston, MA, USA (CTN, PEF); UCSF School of Medicine, San Francisco, CA, USA (JDK, RF); Community-Based Initiative, Ministry of Health, Monrovia, Liberia (MPF); National Institute of Allergy and Infectious Diseases, Monrovia, Liberia (MPF); and A M Dogliotti College of Medicine, University of Liberia, Monrovia, Liberia (MPF)
erichardson@bwh.harvard.edu

This Comment was done with the support of a KL2/Catalyst Medical Research Investigator Training award from Harvard Catalyst/The Harvard Clinical and Translational Science Center (National Center for Research Resources and the National Center for Advancing Translational Sciences, National Institutes of Health Award KL2 TR001100). The content is solely the responsibility of the authors and does not necessarily represent the official views of Harvard Catalyst, Harvard University and its affiliated academic healthcare centers, or the National Institutes of Health.

We declare no competing interests.

1 Kuhn S. Prisoner's dilemma. 2014. https://plato.stanford.edu/entries/prisoner-dilemma/ (accessed Jan 18, 2017).
2 Ferme MC. Hospital diaries: experiences with public health in Sierra Leone. 2014. http://www.culanth.org/fieldsights/591-hospital-diaries-experiences-with-public-health-in-sierra-leone (accessed Jan 18, 2017).
3 WHO. 10 facts on malaria. 2016. http://www.who.int/features/factfiles/malaria/en/ (accessed Jan 18, 2017).
4 WHO Ebola Response Team. Ebola virus disease in West Africa—the first 9 months of the epidemic and forward projections. N Engl J Med 2014; 371: 1481–95.
5 Rosenke K, Adjemian J, Munster VJ, et al. Plasmodium parasitemia associated with increased survival in ebola virus-infected patients. Clin Infect Dis 2016; 63: 1026–33.
6 WHO Ebola Response Team. After Ebola in West Africa—Unpredictable risks, preventable epidemics. N Engl J Med 2016; 375: 587–96.
7 Shultz JM, Cooper JL, Baingana F, et al. The role of fear-related behaviors in the 2013–2016 West Africa Ebola virus disease outbreak. Curr Psychiatry Rep 2016; 18: 104.
8 Rodney W. How Europe underdeveloped Africa. London: Bogle-L'Ouverture, 1972.
9 Farmer P. Social inequalities and emerging infectious diseases. Emerg Infect Dis 1996; 2: 259–69.
10 Rorty R. Contingency, irony, and solidarity. Cambridge: Cambridge University Press, 1989.
11 Richardson ET, Barrie MB, Kelly JD, Dibba Y, Koedoyoma S, Farmer PE. Biosocial approaches to the 2013–16 Ebola pandemic. Health Hum Rights 2016; 18: 167–79.
12 Lewins R. Injection of saline solutions in extraordinary quantities into the veins in cases of malignant cholera. Lancet 1832; 18: 243–44.
13 Richardson ET, Polyakova A. The illusion of scientific objectivity and the death of the investigator. Eur J Clin Invest 2012; 42: 213–15.
14 Bourdieu P, Wacquant LJD. An invitation to reflexive sociology. Chicago, IL: University Of Chicago Press, 1992.

The predicament of patients with suspected Ebola

We appreciate Eugene Richardson and colleagues' framing of the Ebola suspect using the "Ebola suspect's dilemma" heuristic.[1] Nevertheless, we disagree with some data used to inform their argument. For instance, the authors (presumably facetiously) mention that "a rational decision might be to deliberately infect yourself with malaria" on the basis of data showing that patients with plasmodium parasitaemia and Ebola virus disease who received anti-malarial treatment had 20% increased survival compared with a group infected with Ebola virus disease only.[2] In an independent cohort of patients with Ebola virus disease, the inverse was found to be true—mortality was significantly higher in patients with malaria and Ebola virus disease co-infection (66%) compared with patients with Ebola virus disease alone (52%).[3] Thus, the apparent survival benefit has not been reproduced and caution should be exercised when suggesting a potential benefit of malaria in patients with Ebola virus disease. Additionally, the 25% chance of nosocomial transmission of Ebola virus disease cited by the authors is a probable overestimate given that only 3·3% of discharged negative patients returned to Ebola Holding Units in Sierra Leone with Ebola virus disease.[4] Finally, we fully agree with the emphasis of this Comment on the importance of administering intravenous fluid as part of the clinical management of Ebola virus disease. To clarify, fluid loss associated with diarrhoea or shock might occasionally need "injection of saline solutions in extraordinary quantities",[1] as required for some cholera patients. However, as has now been seen in some patients with Ebola virus disease to whom such aggressive fluid resuscitation has been administered, the risk of fluid overload is high, so such risks should be weighed against the potential benefits to appropriately tailor the therapy of a patient with Ebola virus disease.[5]

JvG was coordinating investigator of the European Union-funded Ebola-Tx trial evaluating the use of convalescent plasma as Ebola treatment in Guinea, supported by the Union's Horizon 2020 Research and Innovation Program (under grant agreement 666094). All other authors declare no competing interests.

*Robert Colebunders, Shevin T Jacob, Johan van Griensven
robert.colebunders@uantwerpen.be

Global Health Institute, University of Antwerp, 2610 Antwerp, Belgium (RC); Department of Medicine, University of Washington, Seattle, WA, USA (STJ); and Department of Clinical Sciences, Institute of Tropical Medicine, Antwerp, Belgium (JvG)

1 Richardson ET, Barrie MB, Nutt CT, et al. The Ebola suspect's dilemma. Lancet Glob Health 2017; 5: e254–56.

2 Rosenke K, Adjemian J, Munster VJ, et al. Plasmodium parasitemia associated with increased survival in Ebola virus-infected patients. Clin Infect Dis 2016; 63: 1026–33.

3 Waxman M, Aluisio AR, Rege S, Levine AC. Characteristics and survival of patients with Ebola virus infection, malaria, or both in Sierra Leone: a retrospective cohort study. Lancet Infect Dis 2017; published online Feb 28. http://dx.doi.org/10.1016/S1473-3099(17)30112-3.

4 Arkell P, Youkee D, Brown CS, et al. Quantifying the risk of nosocomial infection within Ebola Holding Units: a retrospective cohort study of negative patients discharged from five Ebola Holding Units in Western Area, Sierra Leone. Trop Med Int Health 2017; 22: 32–40.

5 Uyeki TM, Mehta AK, Davey RT Jr, et al, for the Working Group of the U.S.–European Clinical Network on Clinical Management of Ebola Virus Disease Patients in the U.S. and Europe. Clinical management of Ebola virus disease in the United States and Europe. N Engl J Med 2016; 374: 636–46.

The predicament of patients with suspected Ebola

In their Comment in *The Lancet Global Health*, Eugene Richardson and colleagues[1] criticised the tendency of many analyses of the Ebola epidemic (eg, a WHO report[2]) to ignore that it may be rational for a patient with a fever to avoid an Ebola treatment unit. They use the prisoner's dilemma to explain such non-cooperative behaviour.

The prisoner's dilemma, however, is not the most appropriate analytical framework for this situation. It involves two parties, each with their own interests, while the patient's dilemma might better be understood as a game against nature, ie, without a rational and self-interested opponent. We suggest that the threshold approach introduced by Pauker and Kassirer[3,4] better explains the described phenomenon. The threshold model prescribes a probability of disease at which treatment becomes a better option than no treatment. The threshold is a function of the relative effects of the possible actions and compares the benefit of treating a true Ebola patient against the harm of treating a non-Ebola patient. In this example, exposure to the virus from contact with other (true) Ebola patients represents the harm condition. Using the mortality numbers provided,[1] the benefit is the mortality reduction for true Ebola patients (70·8%–64·3%=6·5%), while the harm is the mortality increase for patients without Ebola (16·1%–0·2%=15·9%). The treatment threshold is calculated as harm/(harm+benefit). Given these data, the treatment threshold is 71·0% (figure). If individuals with suspected Ebola assume that their probability of having Ebola is below this threshold—eg, Richardson and colleagues[1] assume a probability of 50%—the rational behaviour from the individual's point of view is to not seek treatment.

In conclusion, the threshold model[3,4] might explain patients' avoidance of Ebola treatment better and more elegantly than the prisoner's dilemma does.

We declare no competing interests.

*Thomas Mayrhofer, Robert M Hamm, Jef Van den Ende, Iztok Hozo, Benjamin Djulbegovic
tmayrhofer@mgh.harvard.edu

School of Business Studies, Stralsund University of Applied Sciences, 18435 Stralsund, Germany (TM); Massachusetts General Hospital, Harvard Medical School, Boston, MA, USA (TM); Department of Family and Preventive Medicine, University of Oklahoma Health Sciences Center, Oklahoma City, OK, USA (RMH); Institute of Tropical Medicine, Antwerp, Belgium (JVdE); Department of Mathematics, Indiana University Northwest, Gary, IN, USA (IH); USF Program for Comparative Research Effectiveness, Division of Evidence-Based Medicine, Department of Internal Medicine, Morsani College of Medicine, University of South Florida, Tampa, FL, USA (BD); and H Lee Moffitt Cancer Center and Research Institute, Tampa, FL, USA (BD)

1   Richardson ET, Barrie MB, Nutt CT, et al. The Ebola suspect's dilemma. *Lancet Glob Health* 2017; **5:** e254–56.
2   Agua-Agum J, Allegranzi B, Ariyarajah A, et al, for the WHO Ebola Response Team. After Ebola in West Africa—unpredictable risks, preventable epidemics. *N Engl J Med* 2016; **375:** 587–96.
3   Pauker SG, Kassirer JP. Therapeutic decision making: a cost-benefit analysis. *N Engl J Med* 1975; **293:** 229–34.
4   Djulbegovic B, Van den Ende J, Hamm RM, Mayrhofer T, Hozo I, Pauker SG, for the International Threshold Working Group. When is rational to order a diagnostic test, or prescribe treatment: the threshold model as an explanation of practice variation. *Eur J Clin Invest* 2015; **45:** 485–93.

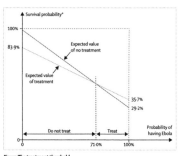

***Figure:* The treatment threshold**
*Survival probabilities are calculated as 100% minus mortality.

The predicament of patients with suspected Ebola

We have concerns about both the accuracy and underlying rationale of Eugene Richardson and colleagues' Comment[1] about the "Ebola suspect's dilemma". The authors quote a nosocomial infection rate of "around 25%" for individuals admitted to Ebola treatment facilities without Ebola virus disease. However, two previous papers document rates of 3%[2] and 7%.[3] In our previous study[4] of over 1000 children admitted to Ebola treatment facilities with suspected Ebola virus disease, only three (0·5%) of 630 children who tested negative were subsequently readmitted with a positive test, all of whom had lost a parent to Ebola virus disease before their first admission; therefore, they were more likely to have acquired Ebola virus disease in the community than nosocomially. Furthermore, the case:fatality ratio of children who were admitted to hospital and were Ebola virus disease-negative was 9% (95% CI 8–12; 66 of 697), similar to previous inpatient mortality rates of children who were negative for Ebola virus disease at Ola During Children's Hospital in Freetown from 2013-2014, prior to the Ebola virus disease outbreak.[5]

By framing the outbreak within the trope of African subjugation or passivity in the face of international colonialists (humanitarian or otherwise), the agency is removed and the sacrifice belittled of the west African health-care workers, such as those who ran the Sierra Leonean Ministry of Health and military facilities in which our study was based.[4] For example, far from "offering little in the way of intravenous resuscitation", the Republic of Sierra Leone Armed Forces provided aggressive parenteral fluid resuscitation from their opening in September, 2014, several months before this protocol was scaled up in internationally run facilities.[6]

Nosocomial transmission rates and mortality rates for children who were Ebola virus disease-negative appear to have been lower than those estimated by Richardson and colleagues, which is testament to the leadership of these Sierra Leonean health-care workers and their commitment to patient care and infection control. By misrepresenting the outcomes achieved by efforts of these west African health-care workers, Richardson and colleagues seem to only bolster the colonial structural determinants that they denigrate.

We declare no competing interests.

*Felicity Fitzgerald, David E Baion, Kevin Wing, Shunmay Yeung, Foday Sahr
felicity.fitzgerald@ucl.ac.uk

Infection, Immunity, Inflammation and Physiological Medicine, UCL Great Ormond Street Institute of Child Health, London, WC1N 1EH, UK (FF); Save the Children, Freetown, Sierra Leone (FF, KW); Save the Children, London, UK (FF, KW); Ola During Children's Hospital, Sierra Leone Ministry of Health, Freetown, Sierra Leone (DEB); Faculty of Epidemiology and Population Health (KW) and Department of Clinical Research (SY), London School of Hygiene and Tropical Medicine, London, UK; and 34 Military Hospital, Republic of Sierra Leone Armed Forces, Freetown, Sierra Leone (FS)

1   Richardson ET, Barrie MB, Nutt CT, et al. The Ebola suspect's dilemma. Lancet Glob Health 2017; 5: e254–56.
2   Arkell P, Youkee D, Brown CS, et al. Quantifying the risk of nosocomial infection within Ebola Holding Units: a retrospective cohort study of negative patients discharged from five Ebola Holding Units in Western Area, Sierra Leone. Trop Med Int Health 2017; 22: 32–40.
3   Fitzpatrick G, Vogt F, Moi Gbabai O, et al. Describing readmissions to an Ebola case management centre (CMC), Sierra Leone, 2014. Euro Surveill 2014; 19: 20924.
4   Fitzgerald F, Wing K, Naveed A, et al. Risk in the "Red Zone": outcomes for children admitted to Ebola holding units in Sierra Leone without Ebola virus disease. Clin Infect Dis 2017; published online March 20. DOI:10.1093/cid/cix223.
5   Ola During Children's Hospital. Data Annual Report 2013 to February 2014. Internal Document, April 2014.
6   Ansumana R, Jacobsen KH, Sahr F, et al. Ebola in Freetown area, Sierra Leone—a case study of 581 patients. N Engl J Med 2015; 372: 587–88.

The predicament of patients with suspected Ebola

Authors' reply

We thank Thomas Mayrhofer and colleagues for offering their threshold model as an explanation for patients' aversion to accessing Ebola facilities during the recent Ebola outbreak in west Africa. We agree that this threshold model provides a rational and more elegant explanation of patients' avoidance of ill-equipped and poorly sanitised holding centres; however, such an explanation was not the goal of our Comment.[1] Instead, we aimed to produce a reductio ad absurdum[2] of rationalist approaches to understanding behaviour during the Ebola outbreak. Our argument was that these approaches reproduce an ideology of individualism that maps poorly onto our understanding of care seeking during the outbreak. By hypostasising individual autonomy and assuming perfect information, rationalist paradigms perniciously normalise the perception that clinical outcomes are a result of patient choice, rather than a result of intentional underdevelopment of health systems[3] coupled with the historical prioritisation by colonial medicine and its legacies (including contemporary humanitarian aid) of containment by isolation.[4] Hence the absurdity of our suggestion that a rational decision for patients with Ebola virus disease might be to deliberately infect themselves with malaria, which Robert Colebunders and colleagues correctly recognise as facetious. Furthermore, our ironic reflections on terms such as "rational" and "superspreader" are a call to recognise and interrogate the categories of thought that are instilled by our training as scientists, clinicians, and public health professionals.[5]

Colebunders and Felicity Fitzgerald and their colleagues also question whether we overestimate the potential for nosocomial Ebola virus transmission. In contrast with the low nosocomial transmission rates that they cite in Freetown, our experience in rural areas—which are so much more poorly resourced than the capital that they are deemed internal colonies[6]—revealed, at times, much less effective infection prevention and control than in the metropole. For example, upon arrival at a rural district hospital in November, 2014, we entered wards crowded with corpses, pools of infectious vomit and excreta, and large amounts of contaminated personal protective equipment. Patients with suspected Ebola virus disease were admitted on clinical grounds because samples, if they were taken, took several days until results were attained; nine (100%) of nine nurses working there contracted Ebola virus disease. Additionally, it was not uncommon for several patients with suspected Ebola virus disease who were vomiting and had diarrhoea to be transported over great distances in a single ambulance. Thus, for the absurdist exercise presented in our Comment, we did not feel that it was far-fetched to posit that a quarter of negative individuals exposed to a similar field of risk could have become infected.

Even so, the purpose of our Comment was to counter the notion that is useful to think in terms of "Ebola suspects" and their ostensible options, while reminding us to question whether the fetishisation of isolation over treatment was "an institutionalised form of non-assistance" that resulted in "a high number of presumably avoidable deaths".[7] As such, our suggestion of the term "PPE [personal protective equipment]-bereft care-nexus" refers to a pragmatic re-description[8] of the "Ebola suspect", in an attempt to provide a more adequate vocabulary for outbreak containment by decolonising humanitarian illusions of bounded subjects.[9] To extend the re-description even further,

we suggest viewing Guinea, Sierra Leone, and Liberia as one large West Africa Ebola Holding Unit (WAEHU) for high-income and upper-middle-income countries around the world, with the implication that the focus on local statistics—including the often cited 70% mortality rate of Ebola virus disease[10]—makes it difficult to distinguish the outbreak from its origins in transnational relations of inequality.[11] A 0% case-fatality ratio in repatriated white American clinicians was achieved outside the WAEHU, which should remind us that such re-descriptions of outbreaks are necessary if we want to integrate power[12] into an understanding of disease dynamics.

We declare no competing interests.

*Eugene T Richardson, Mosoka P Fallah, J Daniel Kelly, Mohamed Bailor Barrie
erichardson@bwh.harvard.edu

Division of Global Health Equity, Brigham and Women's Hospital, Boston, MA 02115, USA (ETR); Partners In Health, Freetown, Sierra Leone (ETR, JDK, MBB); Community-Based Initiative, Ministry of Health, Monrovia, Liberia (MPF); PREVAIL-III Study, National Institute of Allergy and Infectious Diseases, Monrovia, Liberia (MPF); A.M. Dogliotti College of Medicine, University of Liberia, Monrovia, Liberia (MPF); and UCSF School of Medicine, San Francisco, CA, USA (JDK)

1   Richardson ET, Barrie MB, Nutt CT, et al. The Ebola suspect's dilemma. Lancet Glob Health 2017; 5: e254–56.
2   Aristotle. Prior analytics. Indianapolis: Hackett Publishing Company, 1989.
3   Rodney W. How Europe underdeveloped Africa. London: Bogle-L'Ouverture Publications, 1972.
4   Greene J, Basilico MT, Kim H, Farmer P. Colonial medicine and its legacies. In: Farmer P, Kleinman A, Kim J, Basilico M, eds. Reimagining global health: an introduction. Berkeley: University of California Press, 2013.
5   Good BJ. Medicine, rationality and experience: an anthropological perspective. Cambridge: Cambridge University Press, 1993.
6   Zack-Williams B. Diamond mining and underdevelopment in Sierra Leone—1930/1980. Africa Development 1990; 15: 95–117.
7   Ebola: a challenge to our humanitarian identity. A letter to the MSF movement. December, 2014 . http://www.liberation.fr/terre/2015/02/03/parfois-le-traitement-symptomatique-est-ce-neglige-voire-oublie_1194960 (accessed April 1, 2017).
8   Rorty R. Philosophy and social hope. London: Penguin Books, 1999.
9   Mbembe A. On the postcolony. Berkeley: University of California Press, 2001.
10 Agua-Agum J, Ariyarajah A, Aylward B, et al, for the WHO Ebola response team. West African Ebola epidemic after one year—slowing but not yet under control. N Engl J Med 2015; 372: 584–87.
11 Richardson ET, Barrie MB, Kelly JD, Dibba Y, Koedoyoma S, Farmer PE. Biosocial approaches to the 2013–16 Ebola pandemic. Health Hum Rights 2016; 18: 115–28.
12 Mayer J. The political ecology of disease as one new focus for medical geography. Progress in Human Geography 1996; 20: 441–56.

Redescription 6
Not-So-Big Data and Immodest Causal Inference
(Symbolic Reparations)

As an apparatus of the coloniality of knowledge production, epidemiology promotes conservative understandings of health phenomena to the level of common sense. As mentioned previously, this constitutes symbolic violence, since it maintains and reproduces oppressive power structures.

As there are reparations for war and other atrocities, there are also means of performing restitution for symbolic violence. Epistemic reconstitution aims to accomplish this by delinking knowledge production from the modern/colonial matrix of power.[1] Viewing Guinea, Sierra Leone, and Liberia as one large West Africa Ebola Holding Unit or redescribing an Ebola patient as a "PPE-bereft-care-nexus" (as in R3 and R5, respectively) are preliminary attempts at such a delinking. The following audit of the competing paradigms of Big Data and causal inference provides another.

I. Not-So-Big Data and Ebola Virus Disease

> We are at a point in our work when we can no longer ignore empires and the imperial context in our studies.
> —Edward Said, *Culture and Imperialism* (1993)

Background

> Q: What is Big Data?
>
> A: Big Data can be thought of as the information generated by the digitization of social life.

In a 2008 article, science journalist Chris Anderson sounded the first trumpet of the Theory Apocalypse: By promising multidimensional phenomena in full resolution, Big Data is a revolution that will eventually obviate the scientific method. Such a revelatory vision stems from the promise of

> a world where massive amounts of data and applied mathematics replace every other tool that might be brought to bear. Out with every theory of human behavior, from linguistics to sociology. Forget taxonomy, ontology, and psychology. Who knows why people do what they do? The point is they do it, and we can track and measure it with unprecedented fidelity. With enough data, the numbers speak for themselves.[2]

While this annunciation may seem millenarian in its faith that Big Data will apocalyptically overcome theory-ladenness, there are already sobering concerns that the knowledge asymmetries created by the robber barons of surveillance capitalism (Google, Facebook, the US National Security Agency [NSA], etc.) herald new forms of epistemic inequality.[3]

The Blinkered Logic of Protected Affluence
As the authors of a 2016 article titled "Big Data for Infectious Disease Surveillance and Modeling" observed, "The last 15 years have seen the rapid emergence of big data and data science

research, which lies at the intersection of computer science, statistics[,] data visualization"[4]—and, one might add, the blinkered logic of protected affluence. In this latest iteration of "the need to help"[5]—which traces its genealogy to the work of missionaries (i.e., colonizers)[6]—data from electronic health records, surveillance teams, social media, and mobile-phone logs coalesce to provide more accurate infectious disease models and forecasts.

Computational models of epidemics mathematically represent the biology of infectious disease transmission with the aim of forecasting the expected size of an epidemic and the critical level that is needed for an intervention to achieve effective disease control (figure 12).[7] This is sometimes accomplished by generating sets of *simulations* (more on this below) and choosing the one most "consistent with the observed epidemic."[8]

But what does it mean to be consistent with an observed epidemic? Usually, it means that a model provides an accurate prediction of case numbers, human mobility, and transmission dynamics so as to inform containment measures.

During the 2013–2016 Ebola virus outbreak in West Africa, modelers devised a dizzying array of predictions,[9] ranging from the World Health Organization's supposition early on that the outbreak would be contained at a few hundred cases to the Centers for Disease Control and Prevention's estimate of up to 1.4 million cases by January 2015.[10] Interestingly, this latter model was least consistent with the observed epidemic; at the same time, however, it was claimed to be the most useful (as an advocacy tool to muster a robust international response).[11] This is not quite what the renowned statistician George E. P. Box had in mind when he wrote his famous dictum, "All models are wrong but some are useful."[12] Yet when we combine this insight with John Ioannidis's contention that most published clinical

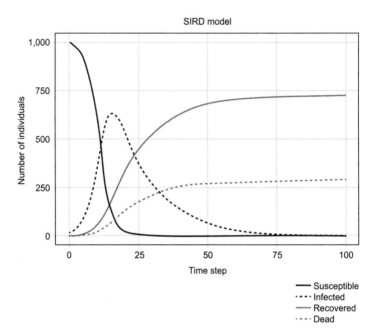

Figure 12
The SIRD model is a simple compartmental model for predicting the growth and decline of an infectious disease outbreak.

research is useless,[13] one starts to wonder whether simulation studies (and other forms of statistical maneuvering that are the currency of epidemiology) have inflated value among high-tier journals as well as policymakers.

Quite the contrary! As will be explored below, the discipline of epidemiology has great utility . . . not as a truth generator,[14] but rather as a means of setting epistemic confines to the understanding of why some groups live sicker lives than others—confines that authorize and sustain protected affluence rather than challenge it.[15]

The Appalling Silence of Mathematical Models (aka Virion Fetishism)

> History will have to record that the greatest tragedy of this period of social transition was not the strident clamor of the bad people, but the appalling silence of the good people.
>
> —Martin Luther King, "Address at the Fourth Annual Institute on Nonviolence and Social Change at Bethel Baptist Church" (1959)

> Any analysis or vision of our world that omits the centrality of Wall Street power, US military policies, and the complex dynamics of class, gender, and sexuality in black America is too narrow and dangerously misleading.
>
> —Cornel West, in *The Guardian* (2017)

Structural violence can be conceived of as a matrix of oppressive forces generated by poverty and steep grades of social inequality, which leads to the frustration of fundamental human needs.[16] Many scholars have probed the structural determinants of the 2013–2016 Ebola virus outbreak in West Africa.[17] The great majority hail from fields—including anthropology, sociology, and environmental science—that are not poised to set the coming episteme, which, if the concerns about Google, Facebook, and the NSA eventuate, may be some form of Big Data coloniality.

A community's episteme can be thought of as the regime of truth to which it abides (see Introduction). As Big Data becomes the means by which scientific truths are sanctioned, that is, as it brings about a change not in method but rather epistemological perspective,[18] the implausible positivist quest to transcend theory-laden investigation may be achieved.[19] In other words, Big Data threatens to confute Anthony Giddens's claim that social scientists "who still wait for a Newton are not only waiting for a train that won't arrive, they're in the wrong station altogether."[20]

Big Data promises significant boons for global health praxis, especially outbreak containment. It seems the Holy Grail of digitizing epidemic response will be to use mobile phone records for contact tracing—leaving aside whether such a seizure of private information is a public good or even ethical—and thus develop predictive models for the spread of disease.[21] Through publication in *Science, Nature,* the *New England Journal of Medicine, Proceedings of the National Academy of Sciences of the United States of America (PNAS),* and other high-impact periodicals that serve to validate the types of discourse that society accepts and makes function as true, these models and their way of parsing the world will become sanctioned, *scientifically* reifying a cognition of infectious disease transmission dynamics where human victims are the agents of spread.[22] In this way, the blinkered logic of protected affluence, which holds that people become sick because a close contact transmitted bits of viral ribonucleic acid (RNA) to their person—not because centuries of predatory accumulation by foreign elites became embodied as hemorrhagic fever—becomes normalized as a commonsense view.[23]

Despite the efforts by honest computational epidemiologists to give caveats about their modeling assumptions, they still rely on ways of validating simulations that not only are insufficient for the way they are used but also harden into common sense a very narrow view of viral transmission dynamics—a view that serves the Global North's protected affluence by depoliticizing understandings of transhemispheric inequality,[24] weakening the disposition of social resistance to such inequality as a result. They do this by translating conservative categories of outbreak phenomena into the doctrinaire language of mathematics and models, mystifying causal forces at the social and historical level.[25] When looked at from the perspective of social medicine[26] and the political economy of health,[27] modelers actually generate sets of *dissimulations*.

Big Data Coloniality

> Conventional anti-colonialism, too, could be an apologia for the colonization of minds.
>
> —Ashis Nandy, *The Intimate Enemy: Loss and Recovery of Self under Colonialism* (1983)

Frantz Fanon revealed how colonial subjects internalize views imposed upon them by their "masters"—what he called "colonial recognition"[28]—and how these views, "along with the structural relations with which they are entwined, come to be recognized (or at least endured) as more or less natural."[29] The same can be said for global health "masters," who tell people the reasons they are sick. Analogous to the way the Zairean client dictator of Cold War neocolonialism Mobutu Sese Seko acted as a "screen between the people and the rapacious bourgeoisie,"[30] master epidemiologists filter out information vital for demonstrating the Global North's complicity in planetary health inequities.

For example, a modeling paper in *PNAS* that claimed to provide a "*complete overview* of the transmission dynamics of the 2014–2015 EVD outbreak in Sierra Leone" (my emphasis) found that Sierra Leoneans had a higher risk of being infected if they (1) lived in a densely populated setting, (2) resided near an Ebola treatment center, (3) had higher cropland coverage nearby, and/ or (4) lived in villages with higher or lower average temperatures than elsewhere.[31] When I brought this study to the attention of colleagues and patients in Sierra Leone, they echoed Linda Tuhiwai Smith's observation of indigenous communities and foreign researchers: "At a common sense level research was talked about both in terms of its absolute worthlessness to us . . . and its absolute usefulness to those who wielded it as an instrument."[32] As such, this "complete overview" of Ebola virus transmission dynamics could also be thought of as an imposition of the settler's gaze.[33]

A counterhegemonic model might compare infected Sierra Leoneans to matched controls in the Global North and find that having (1) been a reserve for slaves, (2) been violently colonized, and/or (3) had most of your nation's wealth looted in the setting of reservoir hosts for Ebola virus (e.g., fruit bats) are associated with Ebola virus infection. Had *this* model informed people's understandings of why they were sick, they might have demanded reparations (i.e., to "recuperate a part of what [had] been stolen from"[34] them) instead of isolation units.[35] With the former, they could have built a health infrastructure capable of containing the outbreak with a small fraction of the deaths recorded.

In another example, Peak and colleagues used Big Data from mobile phone records in Sierra Leone to demonstrate a dramatic reduction in human mobility during a three-day national "stay-at-home" lockdown during the Ebola outbreak.[36] While their "findings" were obvious to most working in the field during the lockdown, the results are problematic for several reasons. First, the false precision of their conclusions—given that mobile phones do not necessarily indicate the precise whereabouts of Sierra Leoneans (since people have multiple phones and share them)[37]—will continue the relegation of qualitative observation to the bins of "soft science"[38] or folklore, depending on who is doing the observing. Second, such an aggregate report of population movements is not useful to those involved in contact tracing;[39] however, the perceived success of digitizing such population movements may lend strength to demands for more identifiable private data, so that contacts can be traced. The application of Big Data for migration analysis without user consent raises crucial questions about the legality of access to such information (especially when the practical value is in question for outbreak containment) and the potential harms of such access.[40] Third, such Big Data was not Big enough to include illicit financial flows (IFFs) from the Global South to their pan-capital depositories in London, New York, Hong Kong, etc.[i] For example,

> African countries received $161.6 billion in 2015—mainly in loans, personal remittances and aid in the form of grants. Yet $203 billion was taken from Africa, either directly—mainly through corporations repatriating profits and by illegally moving money out of the continent—or by costs imposed by the rest of the world through climate change.[41]

As Big Data solidifies "a technocratic monopoly on truth,"[42] one can see the iron cage closing in on global health science.[43] The aura of scientificity[44] provided by terabytes of data crowds out less quantifiable forms of accounting,[45] legitimizing synchronic, apolitical ways of cognizing outbreaks and resultant social suffering.[46]

Which raises the question: are there other models we could conceive of that would be "consistent with the observed

---

i Elsewhere, via a complementary yet nonquantitative exploration of coloniality—small data, in the above paradigm?—we traced how illicit financial flows became embodied as Ebola virus disease in Sierra Leone. R. Frankfurter, M. Kardas-Nelson, A. Benton, et al., "Indirect Rule Redux: The Political Economy of Diamond Mining and Its Relation to the Ebola Outbreak in Kono District, Sierra Leone," *Review of African Political Economy* 45, no. 158 (2018): 522–540.

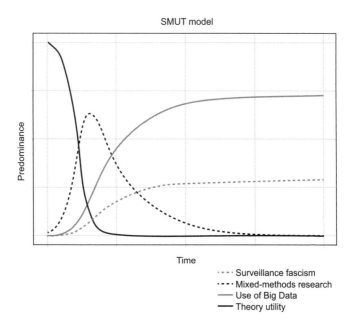

Figure 13
The SMUT model is a simple model for predicting the consequences of unchecked bourgeois reason.

epidemic"?[47] (See figure 13.) The practice of counterhegemonic epidemiology as a form of epistemic reconstitution is not novel;[48] academics and collective health specialists from the Global South have been grappling with it for decades.[49] As an example, Alejandro Cerón has highlighted "the role Guatemalan epidemiologists end up playing in maintaining the quasicolonial social relations of exclusion on which the Guatemalan nation has been built."[50] For the Ebola virus outbreak in West Africa, Fallah and colleagues developed models that quantified poverty as a driver of viral transmission.[51] But such examples are few and far between and still only provide a synchronic structural analysis. Without a historically deep inquiry, one that "successfully" parameterizes (i.e., turns into variables for computational modeling purposes) political-economic forces,[52] unwitting social scientists serve as "mechanisms of normalization [*dispositifs de normalisation*]"[53] for core neoliberal[ii] tenets under the guise of disinterested objectivity (and with the goal of accruing academic capital).[54] Another way of saying this is that they serve as the organic intellectuals of neocolonialism. For future infectious disease outbreaks, a radical reframing of computational epidemiology—and other such "monocultures of the mind"[55] for that matter—is in order, one that transcends the blinkered logic of protected affluence and global health coloniality (Equation 1) to find ways of parameterizing the effects of the Maafa,[56] exploitative colonialism,[57] purposeful underdevelopment,[58] structural adjustment,[59] resource extraction,[60] illicit financial flows,[61] and gender violence,[62] *inter alia* (figure 14).[iii]

$$EBOV\ transmission = f(Maafa,\ Césaire,\ Rodney,\ Kim,$$
$$Curse,\ ILL,\ GV) + \varepsilon \qquad \text{(Eq. 1)}$$

where

EBOV transmission = Ebola virus transmission dynamics
f = a function, possibly nonlinear/nonadditive, of intersecting oppressive forces

---

ii One could substitute *agoramaniacal* (from the ancient Greek words for market and madness) for the term neoliberal.

iii Compelling models linking Africa's current underdevelopment to colonial rule and the slave trade by Nunn and colleagues are a propitious start. N. Nunn, "Historical Legacies: A Model Linking Africa's Past to Its Current Underdevelopment," *Journal of Development Economics* 83 (2007): 157–175.

Maafa = African Holocaust of slavery

Césaire = exploitative colonialism (including neocolonialism)

Rodney = purposeful underdevelopment

Kim = structural adjustment

Curse = resource extraction

ILL = tax evasion and illicit financial flows

GV = gender violence

ε = unobserved bourgeois violence and error

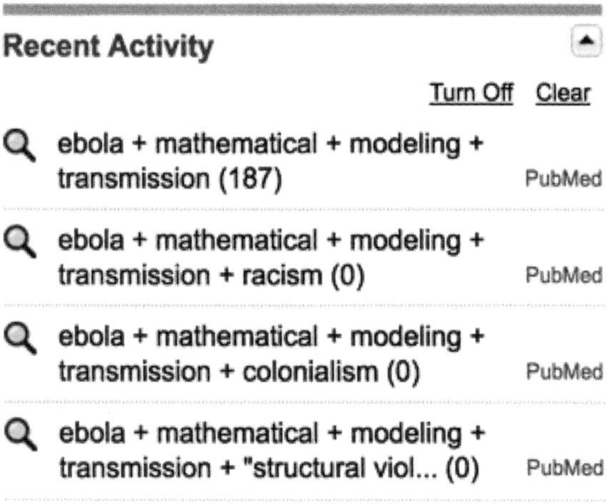

Recent Activity   ▲

                                              Turn Off   Clear

🔍 ebola + mathematical + modeling +
    transmission (187)   PubMed

🔍 ebola + mathematical + modeling +
    transmission + racism (0)   PubMed

🔍 ebola + mathematical + modeling +
    transmission + colonialism (0)   PubMed

🔍 ebola + mathematical + modeling +
    transmission + "structural viol... (0)   PubMed

Figure 14

As part of a not-so-systematic review, I conducted a search in PubMed with the keywords "Ebola + mathematical + modeling + transmission," which yielded 187 results. Only one of the articles included parameterization of models with variables capturing structural violence: M. P. Fallah, L. A. Skrip, S. Gertler, D. Yamin, and A. P. Galvani, "Quantifying Poverty as a Driver of Ebola Transmission," *PLOS Neglected Tropical Diseases* 9, no. 12 (2016): e0004260. This observation was corroborated by individually adding the terms "structural violence," "colonialism," "inequity," "racism" to the keyword string, yielding zero results for each.

II. Immodest Causal Inference

In this way disease is recruited into serving the ideological needs of the social order, to the detriment of healing and our understanding of the social causes of misfortune.

—Michael Taussig, *Reification and the Consciousness of the Patient* (1980)

When we come to you
With hemorrhagic fever
And you isolate us with only ORS,
As to the cause of our illness
An exploration of the local kimberlite pipe[63]
Would tell you more. It is the same reason
We don't polish or cut our diamonds here.[64]

The untreated hypovolemic shock comes,
You say, from an underdeveloped health infrastructure,
And this is also the reason
That 1 in 17 of our mothers will die in childbirth.[65]
So tell us:
Where does this underdevelopment come from?[66]

—"An Ebola Survivor's Speech to a Doctor" (derived from Bertolt Brecht's "A Worker's Speech to a Doctor")

Background

If Big Data's impending "monopoly on truth" described in the previous section represents the Scylla of public health's future epistemic path, then the fetishization of causal inference is its Charybdis.

The causal inference paradigm is a methodological framework based on counterfactual and potential outcomes reasoning, which is coming to dominate the epidemiological literature and pedagogy. By applying "randomized controlled trial (RCT) thinking"—what I like to call the pyrite[iv] standard—to observational data, it allows one to infer the causal status of observed associations by describing how things would change under some hypothetical, well-defined intervention.[v67]

Q: What is Ebola virus illness (EVI)?

A: Medical anthropologist and psychiatrist Arthur Kleinman has described "disease" as a disorder of biology in an individual and "illness" as the resulting polysemic experience of suffering as felt by the patient, caregivers, and society.[68] The coloniality of causal inference in this example hinges on this difference: Ebola virus *disease* allows for causal reasoning, since the inciting event and the outcome are well defined (i.e., Ebola virus infection causes Ebola virus disease in a given individual); however, we are left with a mystification of the structural drivers of suffering (a boon for those in protected affluence). Ebola virus *illness* does not allow for causal reasoning, since Ebola virus illness is not well defined. Instead, it serves as a heuristic maneuver which exposes the conservativity of the causal inference paradigm.

For example, in *The Book of Why: The New Science of Cause and Effect*, computer scientist Judea Pearl uses the graphical chain "Fire → Smoke → Alarm" to demonstrate a simple causal pathway from a fire to an alarm sounding. He writes,

> In science, one often thinks of B as the mechanism, or "mediator,"
> that transmits the effect of A to C. A familiar example is Fire → Smoke

---

iv Fool's gold.

v Note that econometrics has been doing this for a long time, and the techniques, such as instrumental variables, propensity score matching, and regression discontinuity, come from the discipline.

→ Alarm. Although we call them "fire alarms," they are really smoke alarms. The fire by itself does not set off an alarm, so there is no direct arrow from Fire to Alarm . . . This observation leads to an important conceptual point about chains: the mediator B "screens off" information about A from C, and vice versa. . . . For example, once we know the value of Smoke, learning about Fire does not give us any reason to raise or lower our belief in Alarm . . . the variable Fire is irrelevant to Alarm once we know the state of the mediator (Smoke).[69]

If we follow the logic that $Pr(Alarm \mid Fire, Smoke) = P(Alarm \mid Smoke)$—that is, the probability of an alarm sounding in the setting of fire and smoke is the same as the probability in the setting of smoke alone—then for the example Maafa → Ebola virus (EBOV) transmission → Ebola virus illness (EVI), the Maafa is irrelevant to a West African's suffering from Ebola virus illness, since a positive Ebola test tells us what caused the patient's condition (figure 15). In other words, $Pr(EVI \mid Maafa, EBOV) = P(EVI \mid EBOV)$—that is, the probability of suffering from Ebola virus illness in the setting of Ebola virus exposure and the legacies of the Atlantic slave trade is the same as the probability as in the setting of exposure to Ebola virus alone.

Yet Pearl is incorrect about the causal graph. Most modern fire alarms are activated by heat in addition to smoke, and there is thus another causal pathway from fire to alarm (figure 16). This "backdoor path" means the variable Fire is not irrelevant to Alarm, even if we know the state of the mediator (Smoke).

A critical assumption of causal inference is that there be no unmeasured confounding. Physician-epidemiologist Miguel Hernán and colleagues state that we identify confounders through "*a priori* subject-matter or expert knowledge."[70] Yet if, as in the above example, a Turin Award laureate (Pearl) can omit a confounder in the simplest of causal chains, how can we trust more complex phenomena[71]—like whether any of the Maafa's

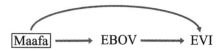

Figure 15

Causal diagram. The presence of the common cause "Maafa" creates an additional source of association between the EBOV (Ebola virus) and the outcome EVI (Ebola virus illness), which we refer to as confounding for the effect of EBOV on EVI. (M. Hernán and J. Robins, *Causal Inference* [Boca Raton: Chapman & Hall/CRC, 2020].) Placing a box around Maafa indicates that one is conditioning on the variable. Without doing so— that is, without including information about the "the history and ongoing effects of atrocities inflicted on African people, particularly when committed by non-Africans . . . specifically in the context of the history of slavery . . . and argued as 'continued to the present day' through imperialism, colonialism, and other forms of oppression" (https://en .wikipedia.org/wiki/Maafa)—one cannot fully explain the causation of EVI by EBOV. Since EVI is not "well defined," however, adherents of the causal inference approach would dismiss it as invalid, hence the conservativity/coloniality of this approach. (S. Schwartz, S. J. Prins, U. B. Campbell, and N. M. Gatto, "Is the 'Well-Defined Intervention Assumption' Politically Conservative?," *Social Science and Medicine* 166 [2016]: 254–257.

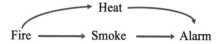

Figure 16
Causal diagram.

legacies were component causes of the Ebola outbreak in West Africa—to "expert knowledge"?[72]

Expert Knowledge, Neocolonial Semiotics, and Global Apartheid

> One central concept in Althusser's writings is ideology. Early on, Althusser had argued that ideology is a "system of representations" governed by rules that serve political ends. . . . ISAs [ideological state apparatuses] reinforce the hegemonic rule of the dominant class by replicating its dominant ideology.
>
> —Michel Lee, "Louis Althusser on Interpellation, and the Ideological State Apparatus" (2015)

Epidemiologist Sharon Schwartz and colleagues have written a brilliant analysis that elucidates the curious conservatism inherent in the causal inference paradigm:

> As the potential outcomes [causal inference] framework becomes branded, disseminated, and implemented, it seems prudent to contemplate the consequences of its adoption for the field. What are the types of questions that are privileged? What are the questions that are left out and what are the implications of their omission? To open the conversation, we pose a provocative claim—that a price may be paid for the clarity that this approach provides, and that price is a conservative articulation of social constructs and a conservative approach to intervention and social change. . . . The determination of what is relevant and plausible is thus presented as an objective, scientific exercise when in reality it is often also a political calculus. By framing as valid only practicable interventions, the potential outcomes approach neglects, discourages, and dismisses more radical change.[73]

I will take their analysis to its Althusserian conclusion and posit epidemiology as an ideological apparatus (like institutions such as churches, schools, universities, schools of public health, families, trade unions, and political parties which reproduce the conditions of the social order)[74] through which practitioners use the causal inference paradigm and unwittingly reproduce the conditions of global apartheid. In essence, I am ironically expressing—as a causal statement—how epidemiology's use of the causal paradigm actually "causes" the conditions this particular epistemic community claims it wants to end.

As an example, I searched PubMed for the most recent article on HIV + causal inference + Africa, since that is an area where I have "*a priori* subject-matter" knowledge. The first relevant paper to come up was the 2018 article "The Impact of ART Initiation on Household Food Security over Time." In this quasi-experiment, Patenaude and colleagues essentially proved that starting HIV therapy in KwaZulu-Natal, South Africa caused an individual's household to become food-insecure, possibly on account of their eating more food as they became healthier on treatment or because they spent household money traveling to and from the clinic. (The authors were able to "control for both omitted variable confounding and reverse causality by identifying quasi-random variation in ART eligibility.")[75]

As Schwartz and colleagues argue, it is difficult to pseudo-randomize variables further upstream in data sets like this,[76] and we are thus left with bright, well-funded computational modelers telling us that we should give food to people who are hungry. But such is the outcome when methods begin to determine the questions we ask.[77] If we really wanted the counterfactual approach to speak to structural determinants, we would end up finding that Black people in South Africa, in order to improve HIV outcomes, would benefit from the well-defined intervention of becoming white (see R8).

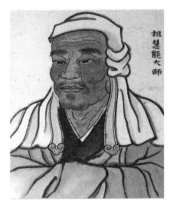

Figure 17
Dajian Huineng, regarded as the 6th Patriarch of the Chan School.

Causal Inference Koan

Some monks were sitting quietly in the garden of a Buddhist monastery on a calm, beautiful day. The prayer flag on the roof started fluttering and flapping in a breeze. A young monk observed: "Flag is flapping." Another monk said: "*Wind* is flapping the flag." The Buddhist master, Dajian Huineng, overhearing the two monks talking, declared: "It is your *minds* that are flapping."

Moral Loopholes and Solidarity

> Mark but this flea, and mark in this,
> How little that which thou deniest me is;
> It sucked me first, and now sucks thee,
> And in this flea our two bloods mingled be;
> Thou know'st that this cannot be said
> A sin, nor shame, nor loss of maidenhead . . .
> —John Donne, "The Flea" (ca. 1590s/1633)

Moral loopholes—that is, schemes via which people avoid ethical behavior they would, under different circumstances, find morally nonnegotiable—are not a contemporary phenomenon. In the poem above, John Donne attempts to convince a fair maiden that since their bodily fluids have already mixed in a flea that has bitten them both, she needn't worry about further consummation sullying her honor. Causal inference actualizes similar moral loopholes (see "Pre-Appendix $e^{i\pi}+6$: Insurrectional Consent Forms" for a more concrete example).

As it achieves further methodological hegemony, causal inference *qua* conservative ideological apparatus will sculpt our moral behavior, since via moral loopholes "identification police" (i.e., those with an exclusive focus on research designs that provide well-defined interventions)[78] like Patenaude and colleagues can choose objectivity over solidarity,[79] resulting in scholarly output that does little to address (and thus contributes to?) human rights deficits.[80] As Iris Young writes, "For if it is a general moral truth that citizens ought to monitor the institutions in which they live and be vigilant lest structural injustice occur within them, then I think it follows that they are culpably negligent if they do not shoulder that burden."[81]

Discussion: Critical Pragmatism and Decoloniality

Imperialism leaves behind germs of rot which we must clinically detect and remove from our land but from our minds as well.
—Frantz Fanon, *The Wretched of the Earth* (1961)

If you stick a knife in my back nine inches and pull it out six inches, there's no progress. If you pull it all the way out that's not progress. Progress is healing the wound that the blow made. And they haven't even pulled the knife out much less healed the wound.
—Malcolm X, TV interview, 1964

Similar to the role philanthropy plays in occulting economic exploitation,[82] the modest improvements in wellbeing offered by global public health science with the right hand disguise what global elites and their looting machines[83] take with the left.[84] For example, the Gates Foundation funded the Institute for Health Metrics and Evaluation (IHME), "the world's premier center for health metrics—the science of measuring and analyzing global health problems,"[85] to the tune of $384 million, and in so doing helped consecrate a discipline that is "ill-suited for considering social quantities as risk factors"[86] for morbidity and mortality. IHME's stated mission is to improve the health of the world's populations by providing the best information on population health, which is somewhat like saying they could have improved the health of American slaves in the seventeenth to nineteenth centuries by counting and reporting how many died from strokes, heart attacks, and malnutrition. There is, in short, no analysis of power.

Their explanations (cited no fewer than 8,500 times) of why some people are sicker than others—high blood pressure, tobacco, and alcohol are their top three[87]—commit hermeneutic injustice (a form of symbolic violence)[88] by authenticating and reifying only downstream risk factors as determinants of morbidity and mortality. In other words, bourgeois-empiricist epidemiology as proffered by groups like the IHME is ideological in the sense that it states reality from the standpoint of dominant interests.[89] It bears repeating: without lending analytical weight to how sociohistorical forces become embodied as pathology,[90] the group unintentionally (since they are no doubt compassionate global health advocates) functions as "transfer mechanisms"[91] for the neoliberal ideology of "predatory individualism,"[92] in essence diverting the public's gaze from legacies of the transatlantic slave trade, colonialism, indirect rule, structural adjustment, and extractive foreign companies (see the Afterword for further critique of their modeling efforts in the setting of COVID-19). More fundamental than questions of credibility,[93] the metrics they use—including the casuistic disability-adjusted life year (DALY)[94]—are social fabrications that masquerade as natural science.[95] To illustrate: If I tell you that a proton is composed of two up quarks and one down quark, no one gets oppressed; however, if I tell you that the Majority World[vi] has worse health outcomes than those in the Global North because of hypertension, tobacco, and alcohol, then I mask the history of exploitation and architected underdevelopment which created these inequitable outcomes in the first place. Furthermore, the main purposes of the DALY are the description/quantification of disease burdens as well as the ranking/choice of interventions. As such, it can be subject to the same critique of conservatism leveled at causal inference's requirement for well-defined interventions.

In this way public health social science colludes with pan-capital in maintaining status quo relations of transnational inequality while vitiating critiques of protected affluence. When the "world's premier" decipherers of global disease burdens reify these particular risk factors, they are more than just "prisoners of the proximate"[96] (i.e., methodologists who understand the determinants of human health in terms of downstream, individual-level risk).[97] Rather, they become the apparatchiki (аппаратчики—Russian for "agents of the apparatus") of global apartheid by decoupling analyses of power from disease dynamics.[98]

---

vi A term coined by Shahidul Alam in 2007.

Epidemiology and Coloniality

As the present epidemiological paradigm (i.e., a focus on the association of risk factors with disease at the individual level)[99] is supplanted by renewed positivistic hope in Big Data and causal inference, global public health scholars should recognize the enduring coloniality—and hence the epistemic struggle[100]—inherent in their work. In order to "interrupt the uncontested flow of inequality"[101] that characterizes the modern world, *conservative analyses of secondary data sets will not suffice*. Just as Sartre concluded that the literary arts may ultimately function as a bourgeois substitute for real commitment in the world, so too may the public health sciences be a diversion from social inquiry as a form of care-knowing.

Q: What is care-knowing?

A: Care-knowing is an approach to social inquiry where care as *disposition* and avoidance of injustice have epistemic significance beyond regulating knowing encounters between individuals.[102]

Redescription 7
Ebola Vaccines and the Ideal Speech Situation
(Border Gnosis)

> Border gnosis as knowledge from a subaltern perspective is knowledge conceived from the exterior borders of the modern/colonial world system . . . conceived at the conflictive intersection of the knowledge produced from the perspective of modern colonialisms (rhetoric, philosophy, science) and knowledge produced from the perspective of colonial modernities in Asia, Africa, and the Americas/ Caribbean.
>
> —Walter Mignolo, *Local Histories/Global Designs: Coloniality, Subaltern Knowledges, and Border Thinking* (2012)

As discussed in the previous redescription, a methodologically individualist approach to global health equity reifies "disease" as a salient and commonsensical phenomenon, enabling causal inference to flourish as an explanatory paradigm. We saw how this approach to parsing health phenomena commits symbolic violence by damming off upstream analyses. By promoting to salience the relational concept of "illness" (see Q&A box on "Ebola virus illness" in R6),[1] on the other hand, we can reforge our common sense and render visible the social machinery of oppression.[2]

In the following redescription, I present qualitative research on Ebola vaccine acceptance conducted as part of the National

Institutes of Health's Partnership for Research on Ebola Virus in Liberia PREVAC study (ClinicalTrials.gov: NCT02876328), as well as conversations with patients I took care of in Ebola treatment centers in both Sierra Leone and the Democratic Republic of the Congo (DRC). When compared to the "scientific" publications of epidemiologists and economists, their Ebola source theories and illness narratives[3] reveal a more relational appreciation of how webs of knowledge/power that stretch back in time and across continents manifest as pathology in human bodies.

Ebola Vaccines and the Ideal Speech Situation[i]

Introduction: The Epidemiologist as Fabricant

The novel *Cloud Atlas* presents a future in which clones known as *fabricants* work as cheap labor in a hypercorporate dystopia.[4] Their minds are stunted via chemical manipulation to prevent them from rebelling or performing radical acts. After 12 years of service, they are promised retirement in Hawai'i, but in actuality they are butchered and recycled as food for other fabricants.

Somewhat analogously, those who seek training in objectivist epidemiology are programmed for a life of unradical (i.e., corporate-friendly) approaches to parsing social phenomena. Their major difference from the fabricant is that they will be fed secondary data sets, which are merely digested bits of the subaltern (insofar as research subjects in the Global South are reaped as academic fodder without any benefit accruing to them).

---

i Parts of this section are adapted from E. T. Richardson, "On the Coloniality of Global Public Health," *Medicine Anthropology Theory* 6, no. 4 (2019): 101–118.

Ebola and the Narrative of Mistrust

They who have put out the people's eyes, reproach them of their blindness.

—John Milton, "Apology for Smectymnuus" (1642)

Early in 2019, researchers from the Harvard School of Public Health published data from a population-based survey in the DRC and concluded that people refused to seek formal medical care or accept vaccines during the 2018–2020 Ebola outbreak because they did not believe Ebola virus was real.[5] The findings were picked up quickly by international news outlets[ii] and helped reinforce a narrative that sufferers of Ebola virus disease (EVD) have their *false* beliefs in conspiracy theories to blame for spread of the outbreak. In the following months, I watched how this narrative of mistrust sedimented as a *cultural* claim of causality among the media, scholars, DRC ministry officials and other responders in North Kivu/Ituri provinces, and the World Health Organization (WHO).

The Social Scientist as Curator

Gather ye facts as ye may.

—Herrick/Richardson, "To the Epidemiologists, to Make Much of Justice" (1648/2019)

My interest, here, is not to refute the authors' reported results—they did gather facts—but rather to expose the epistemic violence

---

ii With the Associated Press reporting, "Researchers said their study showed more precisely how individuals' misinformed views about Ebola were undermining the response and helping to spread the deadly virus." K. Larson, "Study: Many in Ebola Outbreak Don't Believe Virus Is Real," Associated Press, 2019.

such fact-gathering commits (through the analytic omission of diachronic relations of power that determine levels of trust in the postcolony).[6] Nor am I interested in the social construction of facts;[7] as a pragmatist, I accept that there are different ways of parsing phenomena that all vie for epistemic status (that is, for the forefront of consciousness).[8] As wa Thiong'o has taught, "Colonialism imposed its control of the social production of wealth through military conquest and subsequent political dictatorship. But its most important area of domination was the mental universe of the colonised, the control, through culture, of how people perceived themselves and their relationship to the world."[9] This was accomplished through the construction of narratives that produced Africans as racial subjects and sites of savage exteriority, setting them up for moral disqualification and practical instrumentalization.[10] These narratives, which are essentially story technologies invested with (social-)scientific legitimacy,[11] recapitulate the logic of contemporary coloniality.

This redescription aims to demonstrate the ways in which some epidemiologists—like fabricants—have had their moral outlooks stunted by coloniality, which delimits how they gather facts. After discussing counterhegemonic ways of parsing health phenomena, I conclude with ways to delink knowledge production from the colonial matrix of power.

Bourgeois Empiricism and Hermeneutic Injustice
At best, studies like the one conducted by Vinck and colleagues are analytically irresponsible in their collapsing of *trust* and *belief* with health-seeking practices—as well as their insensitivity to the *longue durée*.[iii] At worst, these ahistorical analyses are a form of

---

iii Indeed, for many epidemiologists, *longue durée* would be the name of a parking garage.

neoliberal propaganda that serves to efface the determinants of mistrust that Congolese conspiracy theories are indeed critiquing. Were we to appreciate mistrust as an inclination, a cognitive tendency,[12] or a structured disposition (i.e., habitus) toward eluding depredation—not simply as a rational calculation based on "misinformation"—then its capacity as a mediator in a determinative web of human rights abuses that stretch back in time and link the DRC to distant continents[iv] could rise to the level of common sense.

Instead, however, these studies bound the causal pathway of Ebola transmission to "lack of trust → noncompliant actors → increased risk for EBOV infection" and omit its historical and geopolitical antecedents. In so doing, epidemiologists reify their *mœurs de province* (French for "provincial mores")[v]—which are essentially centuries-old racial hierarchies that have underscored and legitimated the (neo)colonial project—under the guise of objective "empiricism."[vi] In other words, through discursive

---

iv These include the large-scale atrocities committed by King Leopold and Belgium in the late 19th and early 20th centuries, Cold War clientelism and resource theft, and regional genocidal wars whose roots lie deep in the colonial history of ethnic identity construction and mobilization, to name but a few. A. Hochschild, *King Leopold's Ghost: A Story of Greed, Terror, and Heroism in Colonial Africa* (Boston: Houghton Mifflin, 1998); G. Nzongola-Ntalaja, *The Congo from Leopold to Kabila: A People's History* (London: Zed Books, 2013); J. Stearns, *Dancing in the Glory of Monsters: The Collapse of the Congo and the Great War of Africa* (New York: PublicAffairs, 2011).

v The subtitle of Flaubert's *Madame Bovary* (1856). G. Flaubert, *Madame Bovary: Mœurs de province* (Paris: Classiques Garnier, 2014).

vi "The question is no longer the positivist question of whether representation is accurate, copying a reality that is extrasymbolic . . . but what reality is being constructed, by whom, for whom, for what political purpose, and to what political effect." A. Biersack and J. B. Greenberg, *Reimagining Political Ecology* (Durham: Duke University Press, 2006).

hegemony,[13] they prevent structural determination from becoming commonsensical by dominating how people—including both the destitute sick in the Global South and voting citizens and policymakers in the Global North—perceive health phenomena. Such hegemony is also achieved through the domination of authorship by Global North academics: In a follow-up article on conflict and Ebola transmission in the DRC, the same group teamed up with Oxford and IHME to publish an article with zero African coauthors.[14]

As another example, consider the following excerpt from an *Economist* article titled "Death and Disbelievers":

> Many Sierra Leoneans refuse to take the advice of medical experts on Ebola.
>
> When Ebola came to the Kailahun district of eastern Sierra Leone in late May, the government put out a series of messages telling people how to recognize and avoid the disease—among other things by avoiding exposure to victims' blood, sweat, saliva or to dead bodies. Few villagers took any notice. Instead, a string of wild theories is circulating, including suggestions that the government and aid agencies are intentionally spreading the disease. The outbreak highlights a chronic lack of trust between ordinary Sierra Leoneans, their government and the aidgiving Western world. When a burial team including people from foreign charities recently arrived at a village in Kailahun, women and children fled at the sight of their branded vehicles. The men denied they had any bodies to be buried—and chased the team away. Events like these are common.
>
> Some Sierra Leoneans say they fear that the government wants to sell the blood of Ebola patients, or that it will remove patients' limbs for ritual purposes. Others think health workers will inject them with Ebola; or that the ubiquitous chlorine disinfectant spray will give them the disease; or simply that the virus is an invention to help the government bring in donations.
>
> Such beliefs kill. (Anonymous [and Brave] 2014)[15]

Such interpretations kill.

How?

The behavioral inquiries published in *The Lancet Infectious Diseases*, *The Economist,* and other conservative media outlets commit hermeneutic injustice[16] by (1) denying conspiracy theories as valid critiques of the coloniality of power and (2) recycling cultural claims of causality that mystify over 100 years of colonial atrocities and predatory accumulation as explanans.[17] Another way of saying this is that they gather their facts in a manner that serves the interests of protected affluence.

The Ideal Speech Situation

It is as though we have run up a credit-card bill and, having pledged to charge no more, remain befuddled that the balance does not disappear. The effects of that balance, interest accruing daily, are all around us.

—Ta-Nehisi Coates, "The Case for Reparations" (2014)

In his early philosophical work, Jürgen Habermas described the ideal speech situation as a rational exchange of dialogue where unconstrained consensus on truth claims can be achieved.[18] It can be thought of as a utopian version of pragmatism, where truth adjudication is not distorted by domination, ideology, and repression.

If we examine the above narratives of mistrust, we find there is neither consensus nor ideal speech. Rather, in Foucauldian fashion, we can view these discourses as contested sites of power, which help us "make sense of the insidious, often almost invisible nature of ideology today."[19]

From my previous experience taking care of patients and interviewing survivors during the West Africa and DRC Ebola outbreaks, I have come to appreciate such conspiracy theories as a practical logic of engagement with the Maafa (or African Holocaust). As the anthropologist John Clammer notes, "It is in the gaps left by Habermasian reason that in fact real communication and struggle for identity actually take place."[20] Accordingly, these conspiracy theories coalesce with other postcolonial critiques to become truth claims that demand reparations and redistributive justice as interventions—as opposed to (1) bourgeois empiricism (i.e., models of disease causation that obscure sociohistorical forces and "hide behind scientific objectivity to perpetuate dependency, exploitation, racism, elitism, [and] colonialism)"[21] and (2) the crisis caravan (i.e., the flotilla of NGOs and development organizations that move from emergency to emergency, "scattering aid like confetti").[22] By understanding the Maafa as "sedimented situations" lodged inside the body that are waiting to be reactivated,[23] we can reconstitute epidemiology's conservative understanding of EVD "causation."

Mathematized Ideological Systems

"Aid," therefore, to a neo-colonial State is merely a revolving credit, paid by the neo-colonial master, passing through the neo-colonial State and returning to the neo-colonial master in the form of increased profits.

—Kwame Nkrumah, *Neo-colonialism, the Last Stage of Imperialism* (1965)

The unjust gathering of facts is not limited to empirical observation but includes the choice of variables used in epidemiological modeling as well. For example, Bendavid and Bhattacharya used difference models to demonstrate that development assistance for health (DAH, a type of aid) was associated with improvements in health indicators in the countries receiving it.[24] Their results were published in the prestigious journal *JAMA Internal*

Medicine and helped buttress the tenet of neocolonialism summarized by Nkrumah above.

I built a somewhat similar computational model:

$$H_t = \beta_0 + \beta DAH_t + \beta_2 GDPpc_t + \beta_3 Urban_t + \beta_4 TFR_t + \beta_5 IFF_t + \varepsilon_t$$

(Eq. 2)

where *H* is the recent under-5 mortality in a country, *DAH* is the logarithm (log) of the total health aid received from 1970–2008, *GDPpc* is their recent gross domestic product per capita, *Urban* is their percent urbanization, *TFR* is their recent total fertility rate, and ε is an error term. I then added a variable (not included in the *JAMA* analysis) for *Illicit Financial Flows* (IFFs), which can be defined as illegal movements of money or resources from one country to another that reduce the amount of capital and revenue available within a country to develop public services such as health care systems.[25] Subsequent linear regression models demonstrated that *decreases* in under-5 mortality associated with DAH were nearly offset by *increases* in under-5 mortality associated with IFFs. I further found that the log of total health aid was highly correlated with the log of IFFs ($r = 0.65$), raising the question of whether DAH is used to disguise illicit financial flows.

Border Gnosis: Why Are We Sick?

By turning the question this way we allow [sic] the anthropologist's informants the privilege of explicating and publicizing their own criticisms of the forces that are affecting their society—forces which emanate from ours.

—Michael T. Taussig, *The Devil and Commodity Fetishism in South America* (1980)

Intellectuals realize that the masses can do without them and still be knowledgeable: the masses know perfectly well what's going on, it is perfectly clear to them, they even know better than the intellectuals

do, and they say so convincingly enough. But a system of power
exists to bar, prohibit, invalidate their discourse and their knowledge.
—Michel Foucault, "Intellectuals and Power" (1972)

The interviews I conducted with EVD patients, survivors, and
their close contacts provide a counterdiscourse to that employed
by epidemiologists to describe Ebola virus transmission. As discussed in R4, none of these people agreed that using the term
"superspreader" to describe individuals was appropriate. Again,
they focused on corrupt national governments, foreign corporations (e.g., Firestone in Liberia), and the legacy of the Maafa.

In addition, during an Ebola containment campaign in Ituri
Province where my WHO colleagues and I were able to vaccinate
only eight people in a village of more than two hundred, I asked
rural Congolese directly about the mistrust narrative. The replies
were similar to that recorded by the journalist Amy Maxmen:
"People think this is just another thing brought from outside to
kill [us]."[26]

A separate group of individuals who refused the vaccine
agreed that AngloGold Ashanti, one of the largest gold-mining
companies in the region, had helped set the conditions for
the outbreak:[27] "We have nothing to show for all this wealth
underground," a deputy town chief offered. Another chimed
in, "They pay rebels." Such claims have been substantiated: in
a 2010 report, author Adam Hochschild described how Anglo-
Gold Ashanti made "payments to the warlord who controlled
Mongbwalu [in Ituri province] . . . also providing him and his
entourage rides in company planes and vehicles, and a house on
its concession."[28]

After the person voiced the charge that AngloGold Ashanti
paid rebels, I asked the group, "What if I told you that my

university accepted hundreds of millions of dollars from one of the owners of that company?"[vii] "Then they're part of it, too," a part-time miner replied (figure 18).

More often than not, though, my WHO colleagues and I rarely received responses to the question "Why aren't you interested in the vaccine?" (which of course was asked in translation). People often demurred, and when pressed would sometimes offer the conspiracy theories described by Vinck and colleagues.[29] (This reminded me of Evans-Pritchard: "For if Azande cannot enunciate a theory of causation in terms acceptable to us they describe happenings in an idiom that is explanatory.")[30] I might add to this early anthropological insight that "idiom" (i.e., expressed-in-language) includes an interlocutor's habitus. In other words, border gnosis consists of both discursive knowledge and actual practice.

Habitus

In the case of Ebola vaccine acceptance, Kasereka and colleagues reported that there was high community acceptability for the vaccine in the DRC ("72% of unvaccinated community controls would wish to be vaccinated if supply were available").[31] This did not play out in actual practice, though, where I routinely noted less than 20% uptake of individuals who were offered the

---

vii "AngloGold Ashanti mined more than $1.5 billion worth of gold in neighboring Tanzania between 2000 and 2007, but only 9 percent of that money has remained in the country as taxes or royalties. Where do the profits go instead? A good chunk comes to the United States, for even though the company is based in South Africa, its largest single shareholder—hedge fund billionaire John Paulson—lives on the Upper East Side and summers in the Hamptons. He owns 12 percent of the company, and a number of other Americans have shares." Hochschild, "Blood and Treasure."

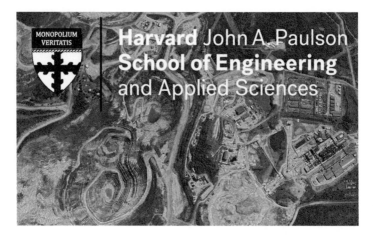

Figure 18
Superspreading nexus. Satellite image of the Kibali gold mine in the DRC superimposed with a revised logo of the John A. Paulson School of Engineering and Applied Sciences (SEAS) at Harvard University (translation from Latin: Monopoly on truth) (image source: Google Earth). Kibali is co-owned by AngloGold Ashanti (45 percent), Barrick Gold Corporation (45 percent) following its merger with Randgold Resources Limited, and Société Minière de KiloMoto (SOKIMO), a state-owned gold mining company (10 percent). In 2015, John A. Paulson, the largest single shareholder of AngloGold Ashanti, donated US$400 million—the largest gift in the university's history—to support SEAS. (J. Sachs, "The Harvard IKB School of Engineering," *HuffPost*, 2016, https://www.huffpost.com/entry/the-harvard-ikb-school-of_b_7518082.)

vaccine. Given the border gnosis highlighted above, we should view this lack of uptake as part of the structured disposition for eluding depredation described earlier.

Harvard Does a Number on the DRC
Between the Harvard School of Public Health committing epistemic violence on one front and the School of Engineering

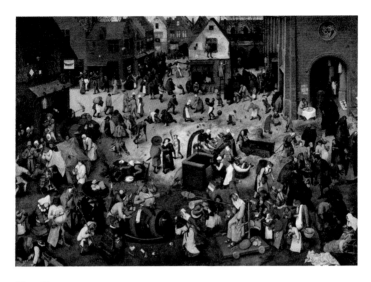

Plate 1

Pieter Bruegel the Elder, *The Fight between Carnival and Lent* (1559). Kunst-historisches Museum, Vienna.

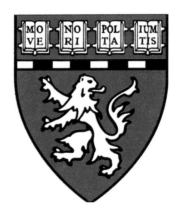

Plate 2

Revised Harvard shield. (Translation from Latin: "Monopoly on Truth.")

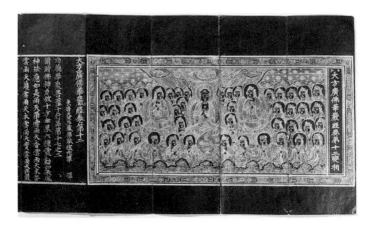

Plate 3

Avataṃsaka Sūtra, vol. 12, frontispiece in gold and silver text on indigo blue paper, mid 14th century.

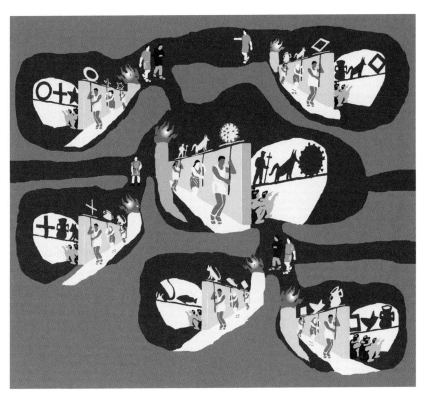

Plate 4

"The Warren," illustration by Lena Gustafson based on a design by Eugene Richardson.

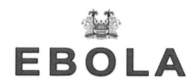

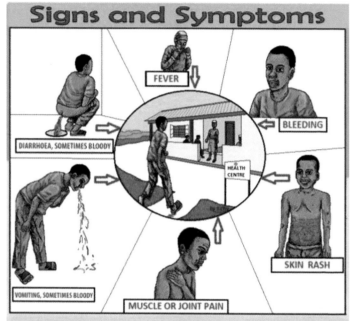

Plate 5
UNICEF poster.

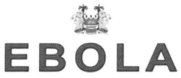

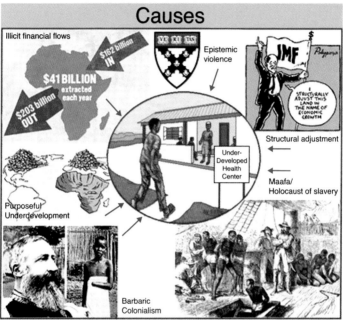

Plate 6
Decoloniality poster.

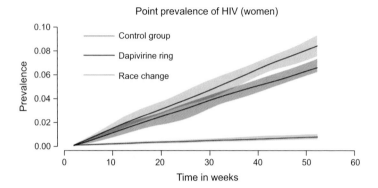

Plate 7

Point prevalence means of HIV for women (lines). Probability of HIV transmission: male to female = 0.300%; female to male = 0.380%. Shaded areas represent 95% of the simulated data. Farthest point to the right marks one-year incidence (Control group = 8.6%; Dapivirine arm= 6.7%; Race change arm = 0.7%). The women's arm starts with 0% prevalence, as being HIV negative was part of the inclusion criteria to enter the study.

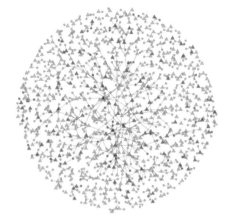

Plate 8

One draw of the network diagram for Control group (50% sample). Blue = susceptible; red = infected; circle = female; triangle = male; lines connecting circles and triangles represent sexual relations.

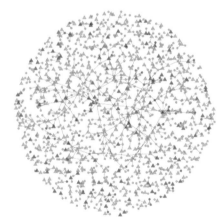

Plate 9

One draw of the network diagram for Dapivirine arm (50% sample). Blue = susceptible; red = infected; circle = female; triangle = male; lines connecting circles and triangles represent sexual relations.

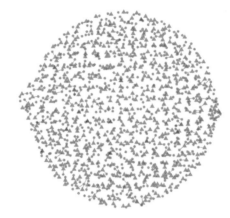

Plate 10

Network diagram for Race change arm (50% sample). Blue = susceptible; red = infected; circle = female; triangle = male; lines connecting circles and triangles represent sexual relations.

reaping the benefits of economic violence on another, how do interested parties begin to address issues of justice? (And this is relevant for other privileged institutions.)

There *are* ways of gathering facts that promote decoloniality: by validating border gnosis like that discussed above as a form of epistemic reconstitution.

Epistemic Reconstitution

Political economists Sara Lowes and Eduardo Montero provide a degree of epistemic reconstitution with their study of medical interventions aimed at eradicating human African trypanoso-miasis (sleeping sickness) in French Equatorial Africa. Utilizing 30 years of archival data from French military archives for five former colonies, including the Congo-Brazzaville, they demon-strate that regions with increased exposure to colonial medi-cal campaigns—characterized by forced lumbar punctures and treatment with aminophenyl arsonic acid (atoxyl), a somewhat effective arsenic compound that left 20% of patients blind—have populations that exhibit lower levels of trust in medicine today.[32] While the authors recapitulate the methodological indi-vidualism and rational agency espoused by Vinck et al., their study is an example of how public health research can begin to parametrize historical and structural forces in shaping popula-tions' dispositions toward medicine and healthcare.

One can hypothesize that a similar dynamic of mistrust was fomented across the Congo River in the Belgian colony, where sleeping sickness suspects were detained in camps (staffed by Catholic nuns) notable for toxic therapy, poor conditions, lack of food, and permanent separation of patients from their families—all under armed guard.[33] Like Alsan and Wanamak-er's excellent study of contemporary mistrust related to the egregiously unethical Tuskegee experiments,[34] these legacies of colonial medicine remind us that mistrust does not form in a vacuum—that is, "cultural" beliefs do not overdetermine health-seeking practices.

Final thoughts

One can note similarities between (1) political scientist Farai Chipato's description of the global aid industry in Zimbabwe, where radical political activists were co-opted into becoming technocratic careerists ("the NGOization of political protest"),[35] and (2) the relegation of political radicals in the United States to schools of public health after the failure of the American left to act as a transformative political-ideological social force.[viii][36]

As fabricants, those relegated to schools of public health have been programmed with bourgeois empiricist (i.e., deradicalized) approaches to parsing health phenomena. As a consequence, they are prone to committing symbolic violence on one front and colluding in economic injustice on the other.[37] By seeing these dual forms of violence as the means by which the modern/colonial racist/patriarchal system[38] continues to operate, we can justify calls for an Epistemic Reformation (see the Conclusion).

---

viii To paraphrase Terry Eagleton, the emancipation which had failed in the streets and factories is instead acted out in nutritional recommendations or logistic regressions. T. Eagleton, *After Theory* (New York: Basic Books, 2003).

Redescription 8
The Race-PrEP Study (Counterhegemonic Modeling)

As posited in R6, if the causal inference paradigm were to be useful in exploring the structural determinants of HIV outcomes in Black people in South Africa, we would end up finding that such individuals would benefit from the well-defined intervention of becoming white.

The following research article shows what this might look like as a computational modeling exercise. It uses a form of (R)hetoric[1] known as R code. R is a programming language that allows individuals, or groups of individuals, to depoliticize complex, historical phenomena into bits amenable to computational manipulation. As a tool of coloniality and a vehicle for symbolic violence, R is mostly used to generate the *dissimulations* described in R4 and R6.

(The (R)hetoric I indited to accomplish the task can be found in Pre-Appendix ـم.)

Modeling Race Change vs. Dapivirine Pre-exposure Prophylaxis in South African Women at High Risk for HIV Infection: The Race-PrEP Study

Eugene T. Richardson, MD, PhD[a][b]

Abstract

Background: The low efficacy of oral pre-exposure prophylaxis (PrEP) in high-risk African women suggests that biomedical interventions are not a total solution to the prevention of HIV infection since they presuppose unconstrained individual agency and medicalize a disease-free state. Changing race could provide a solution.

Methods: Utilizing inputs from previous PrEP studies and meta-analyses, as well as empirical data from sub-Saharan Africa, I developed a stochastic network model to simulate HIV transmission through sexual networks, using the separable temporal exponential random graph model (STERGM) framework. I then simulated a clinical trial of 6,000 South African women at high risk for HIV acquisition from heterosexual intercourse using VOICE study inclusion criteria. One thousand five hundred Black women were turned into white women,

Correspondence: Eugene T. Richardson, MD, PhD. Harvard Medical School, Department of Global Health and Social Medicine, 641 Huntington Avenue, Boston, MA 02115, Eugene_Richardson@hms.harvard.edu

a. Department of Global Health and Social Medicine, Harvard Medical School, Boston, USA
b. Department of Medicine, Brigham and Women's Hospital, Boston, USA

another 1,500 Black women were turned into white women and also received a dapivirine ring, 1,500 Black women received a monthly dapivirine ring as PrEP but stayed Black, and 1,500 acted as controls (i.e., received neither race treatment nor biomedical intervention).

Results: If Black women used the dapivirine ring, then their yearly HIV incidence would decrease from a baseline of 8.6% to 6.7%. The models predict 129 HIV infections in the race control group and 101 in the PrEP (dapivirine) arm (relative risk [RR] = 0.775, 95% CI: 0.603–0.996). If Black women turned white, yearly HIV incidence would decrease from 8.6% to 0.7% (RR = 0.085, 95% CI: 0.046–0.157). Adding dapivirine to race change did not significantly reduce incidence further.

Conclusions: If Black women at high risk for HIV acquisition turned white and accrued the associated structural benefits, they could reduce their HIV incidence twelvefold, even as compared to biomedical interventions.

Keywords: coloniality, race, HIV, pre-exposure prophylaxis, sexual networks, stochastic simulation

Word count: 1485

＊

If we had job opportunities, this blesser[i] thing would go away.

—Nonhle Khomo, *Tonic-Vice* (2016)[2]

Introduction
Pre-exposure Prophylaxis
Despite decades of social science research, it has become clear that efforts to end the HIV epidemic have been hampered by insufficient attention to structural influences on risk of infection.[3] Indeed, the effective methods recognized by the scientific community to prevent new HIV infections remain limited to biomedical strategies.[4] Male circumcision and treatment as prevention (TasP) are currently being rolled out as evidence-based interventions.[5] Adding to this toolbox of possibilities, there has been a groundswell of research dollars aimed at chemoprophylaxis in non-infected individuals. One modality in particular, oral preexposure prophylaxis (PrEP),

---

i Another term for sugar-daddy.

has generated successful prevention outcomes for men who have sex
with men (MSM) and serodiscordant couples;[6] however, the strategy
showed no preventive benefit in two
large randomized controlled trials
(RCTs) of African women at high
risk for infection.[7] There are three
major theories as to why PrEP failed
in these trials: (1) the women were
non-adherent because the random-
ized/placebo nature of the trials pro-
moted distrust and lack of confidence
in the pills they were receiving;[8] (2)
PrEP efficacy is undermined by the
vaginal microbiome;[9] (3) the women
were non-adherent because of the
economic, political, and cultural factors that coalesce as institutional
racism and influence women's abilities to adhere to medical regimens.[10]
The first two hypotheses are challenged by evidence from Partners-
PrEP, a randomized placebo trial that
showed PrEP efficacy and adherence
in women in serodiscordant relationships.[11] The third has been compel-
lingly theorized,[12] but there is limited
empiric evidence in relation to PrEP.

In attempting to offer a "user-
controlled" intervention, the prescript
of daily pill-taking overlooks gender
differences in power and resources
that can limit the effectiveness of
such an approach.[13] As Hanna and
Kleinman contend, "When structural

violence is overlooked, agency is
often overestimated."[14] Young women
are often not able to discuss HIV or
negotiate partner testing and condom
use due to concerns about domestic
violence, preserving the partnership,
or economic loss.[15]

Concerns about the burden of
adherence of daily pill-taking have
led to the development of long-
acting products (e.g., injectables and
insertable devices). One example of
the latter is the dapivirine ring, an
intra-vaginal form of PrEP inserted
monthly which obviates daily pill-
taking. In randomized controlled
clinical trials, the dapivirine ring
showed a 27%[16] and 31%[17] protective
benefit in high-risk women compared
to placebo; however, in both trials, the
ring failed to reduce HIV incidence in
women less than 21 years of age.

Hypothesis

The failure of oral PrEP and limited
efficacy of vaginal PrEP in high-
risk African women suggests that
biomedical interventions are not
a total solution for the prevention
of infection since they presuppose
unconstrained individual agency and
medicalize a disease-free state.[18] The
working hypothesis in the following
simulations is that changing from
Black to white will help women negotiate the structural factors that lead

to HIV acquisition (see figure 19 for the Directed Acyclic Graph or DAG). I model the effect this might have on HIV incidence amongst African women at high risk for HIV.

Methods

Utilizing inputs from previous PrEP studies[19] and meta-analyses,[20] as well as empirical data from South Africa,[21] I developed stochastic network models to simulate HIV transmission through sexual networks, using the separable temporal exponential random graph model (STERGM) framework[22] to predict the probability of partnerships forming and dissolving. The models accounted for gender, HIV status, heterogeneity in transmission rates, partnership duration, coital frequency, partner choice, concurrency, and death rates. Models were built using the EpiModel package[23] in R (version 3.6.1).

I then simulated a clinical trial of 6,000 South African women at high risk for HIV acquisition from heterosexual intercourse using VOICE study inclusion criteria.[24] One thousand five hundred Black women were turned into white women, another 1,500 Black women were turned into white women and also received a dapivirine ring, 1,500 Black women received a monthly dapivirine ring as PrEP but stayed Black, and 1,500 acted as controls (i.e., received neither race treatment nor biomedical intervention). By initializing the models with data from other PrEP studies, I accounted for the behavioral conditioning that women involved in PrEP trials receive (as a result of HIV prevention counseling). Transmission was modeled in weekly time increments over a one-year period.

For the number of concurrent partnerships, I used the degree distributions for high risk South African men and women reported by Delva and colleagues.[25]

Results/Discussion

If the Black women used the dapivirine ring, then their yearly HIV incidence would decrease from a baseline of 8.6% to 6.7% (figure 20). The 8.6%

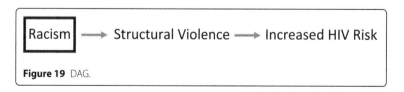

Figure 19 DAG.

incidence modeled in the control arm is similar to data on high-risk subgroups of South African women from the VOICE trial, where incidence was nearly 10% among unmarried women under 25 years of age.[26] The models predict 129 HIV infections in the race control group and 101 in the PrEP (dapivirine) arm (relative risk [RR] = 0.775, 95% CI: 0.603–0.996).

If Black women turned white, yearly HIV incidence would decrease from 8.6% to 0.7% (RR = 0.085, 95% CI: 0.046–0.157). Adding dapivirine to race change did not significantly reduce incidence further.

Figure 21 shows a network diagram of the control group. Figures 22 and 23 show network diagrams of the dapivirine arm and the race change arm, respectively.

Conclusions

Since randomized trials comparing chemical interventions to structural prevention are rarely performed, mathematical models of HIV/AIDS can summarize known epidemiology, treatment, and prevention data with pragmatic results for both policy and further research.[27] These results demonstrate that if Black women at high risk for HIV acquisition turned white and accrued the associated structural benefits, they could reduce their HIV incidence twelvefold.

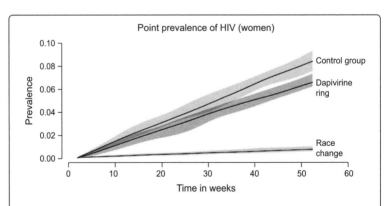

Figure 20 Point prevalence of HIV for women (lines). Probability of HIV transmission: male to female = 0.300%; female to male = 0.380%. Shaded areas represent 95% of the simulated data. Farthest point to the right marks one-year incidence (Control group = 8.6%; Dapivirine arm= 6.7%; Race change arm = 0.7%). The women's arm starts with 0% prevalence, as being HIV negative was part of the inclusion criteria to enter the study.

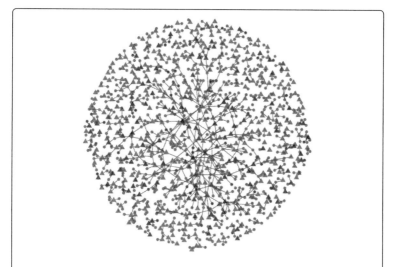

Figure 21 One draw of the network diagram for Control group (50% sample). Blue (light gray) = susceptible; red (dark gray) = infected; circle = female; triangle = male; lines connecting circles and triangles represent sexual relations. (See plate 8 for color.)

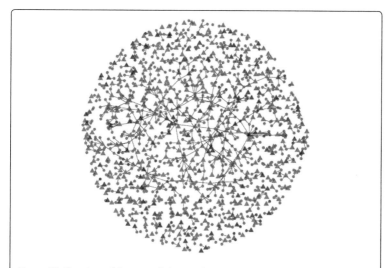

Figure 22 One draw of the network diagram for Dapivirine arm (50% sample). Blue (light gray) = susceptible; red (dark gray) = infected; circle = female; triangle = male; lines connecting circles and triangles represent sexual relations. (See plate 9 for color.)

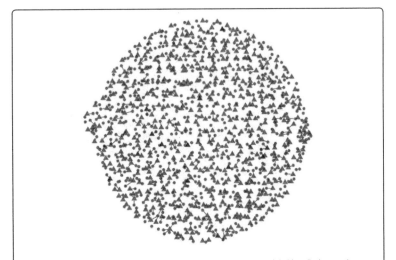

Figure 23 Network diagram for Race change arm (50% sample). Blue (light gray) = susceptible; red (dark gray) = infected; circle = female; triangle = male; lines connecting circles and triangles represent sexual relations. (See plate 10 for color.)

Limitations

Departing from imperious irony, it is, of course, incoherent to imagine people switching their race (in order to measure the treatment effect of race) if race is conceived of as an intersubjective construct of social practices, institutions, norms, expectations, etc.[28] Rather, race change serves as a heuristic device that can be used to demonstrate the conservativity inherent in causal inference as a paradigm for understanding global health inequity; it is the only "well-defined" intervention that could sum up so many structural pathways of harm.[29] We should be wary of causal inference's growing hegemony as an epidemiologic paradigm.

Pre-Appendices

This book has experimented with form for a variety of reasons:[1]

١. To offer a critique of coloniality without being bound by its terms of reference.[2]

2. To blur the boundaries between manifesto and scholarly pseudomonograph, and therefore to unsettle the tradition of academic rent-seeking.[i]

٣. To subvert the means by which "scientific" journal articles convey authority through an Intro-Methods-Results-Conclusion format by co-opting it for alternative knowledge ecologies.

---

i "Rent Seeking—The feature of feudalism that is anathema to both capitalists and socialists, it consists in the capacity to generate value by making a resource—be it land or labor—less rather than more productive. This condition is made possible by the monopoly nature of ownership, which in turn allows 'rent' to be charged prior to any use of the resource. As long as potential users have no alternative but to go through the owner to get what they want, rents can be charged. In the post-truth condition, expertise—and perhaps academic knowledge more generally—is regarded as a form of rent-seeking." S. Fuller, *Post-Truth: Knowledge as a Power Game* (London: Anthem Press; 2018).

四. For the present section, so that people may actually read it (since appendices that follow the Conclusion are often passed over).

Pre-Appendix 五: Race-PrEP R code

```
##——setup——————————————————————
library(EpiModel)

##———network structure————————————
num.m1 <- 1500
num.m2 <- 1070
nw <- network.initialize(n = num.m1 + num.m2,
  bipartite = num.m1,
  directed = FALSE)
nw

##——degree distributions——————————
deg.dist.m1 <- c(0, 0.79, 0.13, 0.05, 0.03)
deg.dist.m2 <- c(0, 0.55, 0.19, 0.12, 0.14)

check_bip_degdist(num.m1, num.m2,
  deg.dist.m1, deg.dist.m2)

##————model parameters————————————
formation <- ~ edges + b1degree(1:2) + b2degree(1:2)
target.stats <- c(1980,1185,195,589,203)

dissolution <- ~ offset(edges)
duration <- 52
coef.diss <- dissolution_coefs(dissolution, duration,
d.rate = 0.0067)

##——Control model fit——————————————
est <- netest(nw,
  formation,
  target.stats,
  coef.diss,
  edapprox = TRUE)
```

```
##————model diagnostics————
mcmc.diagnostics(est$fit, vars.per.page = 5)

dx <- netdx(est, nsims = 5, nsteps = 52,
nwstats.formula = ~ edges + b1degree(0:3) +
b2degree(0:3))
dx
par(mfrow = c(1, 1), mar = c(1, 1, 1, 1))
plot(dx)

##————model fit (transmission rate for LIC's, without
CSE, Boily 2009)————————
param <- param.net(inf.prob = 0.003, inf.prob.m2 =
0.0038, act.rate=2.5)

##————————(20% prevalence for male arm)————————
init <- init.net(i.num = 0, i.num.m2 = 214, status.rand
= FALSE)

##————————(2.5% prevalence for race change male
arm)————————
init2 <- init.net(i.num = 0, i.num.m2 = 27, status.rand
= FALSE)

##————————————————————————————————
control <- control.net(type = "SI",
  nsims = 100,
  nsteps = 52,
  nwstats.formula = ~ edges +
    b1degree(0:4) +
    b2degree(0:4),
  save.network = TRUE)

##————summary————————————————————
sim1 <- netsim(est, param, init, control)

##————Race change degree distributions————————
deg.dist.m1.3 <- c(0.23,0.73,0.03,0.01,0)
deg.dist.m2.3 <- c(0.14,0.67,0.12,0.04,0.03)
```

```
check_bip_degdist(num.m1, num.m2,
   deg.dist.m1.3, deg.dist.m2.3)

##————model parameters——————
formation.3 <- ~ edges + b1degree(1:2) + b2degree(1:2)
target.stats.3 <- c(1230, 1095, 45, 717, 128)

dissolution.3 <- ~ offset(edges)
duration.3 <- 52
coef.diss.3 <- dissolution_coefs(dissolution=dissolut
ion.3, duration=duration.3,
   d.rate = 0.0067)

##————Race change model fit——————
est3 <- netest(nw,
   formation=formation.3,
   target.stats=target.stats.3,
   coef.diss=coef.diss.3,
   edapprox = TRUE)

##————model diagnostics——————
mcmc.diagnostics(est3$fit, vars.per.page = 5)

dx3 <- netdx(est3, nsims = 5, nsteps = 52,
   nwstats.formula = ~ edges + b1degree(0:3) +
   b2degree(0:3))
dx3

plot (dx3)

##————Race change model simulation————
sim3 <- netsim(est3, param, init2, control)

##————27% Dapvirine ring protection model
simulation——————
param.5 <- param.net(inf.prob = 0.00219, inf.prob.m2 =
0.0038, act.rate=2.5)
sim9 <- netsim(est, param.5, init, control)

##————1-year incidence summaries——————
summary(sim1, at = 52)
```

```
summary(sim9, at = 52)
summary(sim3, at = 52)

##————Point prevalence
plots—————————————————
par(mfrow = c(1, 1), mar = c(5, 5, 5, 5))
plot(sim1, y = "i.num", popfrac=TRUE,
   qnts = .95, mean.col = "black", qnts.col =
   "steelblue",
   ylim=c(0, 0.10), xlim=c(0,60),
   main="Point prevalence of HIV (women)", xlab="Time in
   weeks")
plot(sim9, y = "i.num", popfrac=TRUE, mean.col =
"black",
   qnts = 0.95, qnts.col = "firebrick", add = TRUE)
plot(sim3, y = "i.num", popfrac=TRUE, mean.col =
"black", qnts = 0.95,
   qnts.col = "green",add = TRUE)
legend(x=0, y=0.12, c("Control group",
     "Dapivirine ring",
     "Race change"), lty = 1, y.intersp=0.5,
   col = c("steelblue", "firebrick", "green"), lwd = 3,
   bty = "n", cex = 1.4)

##————network plots of 50% of sample [control]
———————————————

num.m1.4 <- 750
num.m2.4 <- 535
nw.4 <- network.initialize(n = num.m1.4 + num.m2.4,
   bipartite = num.m1.4,
   directed = FALSE)

deg.dist.m1 <- c(0, 0.79, 0.13, 0.05, 0.03)
deg.dist.m2 <- c(0, 0.55, 0.19, 0.12, 0.14)

check_bip_degdist(num.m1.4, num.m2.4,
   deg.dist.m1, deg.dist.m2)

target.stats.4 <- c(990,593,98,294,102)
```

```
est4 <- netest(nw=nw.4,
   formation,
   target.stats=target.stats.4,
   coef.diss,
   edapprox = TRUE)

init.4 <- init.net(i.num = 0, i.num.m2 = 107, status.
rand = FALSE)

control.4 <- control.net(type = "SI",
   nsims = 100,
   nsteps = 52,
   nwstats.formula = ~ edges +
      b1degree(0:4) +
      b2degree(0:4),
   save.network = TRUE)

sim4 <- netsim(est4, param, init=init.4,
control=control.4)

##------Race change-----------
deg.dist.m1.3 <- c(0.23,0.73,0.03,0.01,0)
deg.dist.m2.3 <- c(0.14,0.67,0.12,0.04,0.03)

check_bip_degdist(num.m1.4, num.m2.4,
   deg.dist.m1.3, deg.dist.m2.3)

target.stats.5 <- c(615,548,23,358,64)

est5 <- netest(nw=nw.4,
   formation=formation.3,
   target.stats=target.stats.5,
   coef.diss=coef.diss.3,
   edapprox = TRUE)

init.5 <- init.net(i.num = 0, i.num.m2 = 14, status.
rand = FALSE)

sim5 <- netsim(est5, param, init=init.5,
control=control.4)
```

```
##──Dapivirine──────
sim20 <- netsim(est4, param.5, init=init.4,
control=control.4)

##──────network plots───────
get_msim <- function(x, at)
{ which.min(abs(as.numeric(x$epi$i.num[at, ]) -
  mean(as.numeric(x$epi$i.num[at, ]))))}
med.si4 <- get_msim(sim4, 52)
med.si5 <- get_msim(sim5, 52)

par(mfrow = c(1, 1), mar = c(0,0,2,0))

plot(sim4, type = "network", at = 52,
  sims = "mean", col.status = TRUE, shp.bip =
  "triangle",
  mode = "fruchtermanreingold",
  object.scale=0.006)

plot(sim5, type = "network", at = 52,
  sims = "mean", col.status = TRUE, shp.bip =
  "triangle",
  mode = "fruchtermanreingold", object.scale=0.006)

plot(sim20, type = "network", at = 52,
  sims = "mean", col.status = TRUE, shp.bip =
  "triangle",
  mode = "fruchtermanreingold",
  object.scale=0.006)
```

Pre-Appendix 2: The Nkrumahtic Oath[ii]

I swear to fulfill, to the best of my ability and judgment, this
covenant:

---

ii Modeled on Louis Lasagna's "Modern Hippocratic Oath." L. Lasagna,
"Modern Hippocratic Oath," 1964, http://guides.library.jhu.edu/content
.php?pid=23699&sid=190964.

I will respect the hard-won gains of the despised classes and duly affirm that my way of seeing the world admits others.

I appreciate that "what makes ideas 'real' is the system of knowledge, the formations of culture, and the relations of power in which these concepts are located."[3]

I will apply, for the benefit of the anti-Eurocentric, all measures required to democratize knowledge.

I will remember that there is art to social inquiry, and that I should gather facts always with a view toward justice.

I am aware of the continuities between the colonial past and current racialized and hierarchical world order.

I am committed to "pluriversalism as opposed to the failing universalism predicated on Euro-American hegemonic epistemologies."[4]

I hold that "some people can rightly claim that their individual interactions with other people are impeccable, and that at the same time they contribute a great deal to the production and reproduction of structural injustice because of the social position they occupy and the actions they take within it."[5]

I recognize that exploitative socioeconomic relations are foundational to the social order, and these have a fundamental shaping effect on social ideation.[6]

I will not be ashamed to say "I know not," since structural humility is a virtue.[7]

I affirm that "Racial capitalism is the equivalent of a giant necropolis. It rests on the traffic of dead and human bones."[8]

I will challenge "the ideological distortions built into mainstream perspectives and, insofar as possible, [compel] their adherents to respond."[9]

I will remember that I remain a member of society, with special obligations to all my fellow human beings, those sound of mind and body as well as the infirm.

I hold that the Global North represents the most morally stunted civilization in history, given widespread global poverty and suffering compared with our capacity to end it.[10]

I understand that the "prognosis is in the hands of those who are prepared to shake the worm-eaten foundations of the edifice."[11]

If I do not violate this oath, may I enjoy life and art, respected while I live and remembered with affection thereafter. May I always act so as to preserve the finest traditions of my calling and may I long experience the joy of healing those who seek my help.

Pre-Appendix ٣: Disruptive Social Media

On July 28, 1999 two teenage stowaways named Yaguine Koita and Fodé Tounkara froze to death in the wheel bay of a Sabena Airlines flight from Conakry, Guinea to Brussels, Belgium. Their bodies were discovered five days later with the following letter (translated here from French):

Excellencies, Messrs. members and officials of Europe,

We have the honorable pleasure and the great confidence in you to write this letter to speak to you about the objective of our journey and the suffering of us, the children and young people of Africa.

But first of all, we present to you life's most delicious, charming and respected greetings. To this effect, be our support and our assistance. You are for us, in Africa, those to whom it is necessary to request relief. We implore you, for the love of your continent, for the feeling that you have towards your people and especially for the affinity and love that you have for your children whom you love for a lifetime. Furthermore, for the love and meekness of our creator God the omnipotent one who gave you all the good experiences, wealth and ability to ably construct and organize your continent to become the most beautiful one and most admirable among the others.

Messrs. members and officials of Europe, we call out for your solidarity and your kindness for the relief of Africa. Do help us, we suffer enormously in Africa, we have problems and some shortcomings regarding the rights of the child.

In terms of problems, we have war, disease, malnutrition, etc. As for the rights of the child in Africa, and especially in Guinea, we have too many schools but a great lack of education and training. Only in the private schools can one have a good education and good training, but it takes a great sum of money. Now, our parents are poor and it is necessary for them to feed us. Furthermore, we have no sports schools where we could practice soccer, basketball or tennis.

This is the reason, we, African children and youth, ask you to create a big efficient organization for Africa to allow us to progress.

Therefore, if you see that we have sacrificed ourselves and risked our lives, this is because we suffer too much in Africa and that we need you to fight against poverty and to put an end to the war in Africa. Nevertheless, we want to learn, and we ask you to help us in Africa learn to be like you.

Finally, we appeal to you to excuse us very, very much for daring to write this letter to you, the great personages to whom we owe much respect. And do not forget it is to you whom we must lament about the weakness of our abilities in Africa.

Written by two Guinean children,
Yaguine Koita and Fodé Tounkara[12]

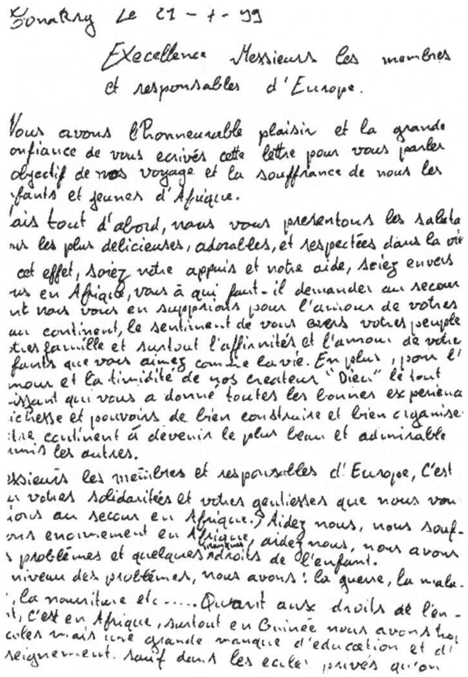

Conakry le 21 - 1 - 99

Excellence Messieurs les membres
et responsables d'Europe.

Vous avons l'honneurable plaisir et la grande
onfiance de vous ecrivés cette lettre pour vous parler
objectif de nos voyage et la souffrance de nous les
fants et jeunes d'Afrique.
'ais tout d'abord, nous vous presentons les saluta
ns les plus delicieuses, adorables, et respectées dans la vie
cet effet, soiez votre appuis et votre aide, soiez envers
us en Afrique, vous à qui faut-il demander au secour
nt nous vous en suppliants pour l'amour de votres
au continent, le sentiment de vous avers votres peuple
tres famille et surtout l'affinités et l'amour de votre
fants que vous aimez comme la vie. En plus, pour l'
mour et la timidité de nos createur "Dieu" le tout
issant qui vous a donné toutes les bonnes experienc
ichesse et pouvoirs de bien construire et bien organise
tre continent á devenir le plus beau et admirable
rmis les autres.
ssieurs les membres et responsables d'Europe, C'est
n votres solidarités et votres gentiesses que nous vou
ions au secour en Afrique. Aidez nous, nous souf-
ons enormement en Afrique, aidez nous, nous avons
s problèmes et quelques droits de l'enfant.
niveau des problèmes, nous avons: la guerre, la mala
, la nourriture etc..... Quant aux droits de l'en-
t, c'est en Afrique, surtout en Guinée nous avons bea
coles mais une grande manque d'education et d'
seignement. sauf dans les ecoles privés qu'on

Figure 24
Epistle.

Second E-pistle to the Leisure Class

Despite its association with early Christianity, the epistolary genre was pioneered in Egypt from around the 25th century Before the Common Era (BCE). The following e-pistle (translated from Mandinka) was sent from the Gmail account of one of two West African migrants who drowned in August 2018 after their boat capsized in the Mediterranean Sea (previously known as Wadj-Ur or 𓇅𓅨𓈗 in Ancient Egyptian):

Excellencies, Paramount members and officials of Europe,

We have the honorable pleasure and the great confidence in you to write this letter to speak to you about the objective of our journey and the suffering of us, the children and young people of Africa.

But first of all, we present to you life's most delicious, charming and respected greetings. To this effect, be our support and our assistance. You are for us, in Africa, those to whom it is necessary to request relief, since it is you who have not only extracted humans from our continent, but much of our resources as well. We implore you, for the love of your continent, whose wealth was built on African exploitation. Furthermore, for the love and meekness of the creator God who you invented and with whom you proceeded to violently proselytize us, committing epistemicide.

Paramount members and officials of Europe, we call out for you to recognize the words of our uncle Jean-Bertrand Aristide, who said "We're asking you to acknowledge what you've stolen, that your countrymen have stolen during the process of colonization. If you truly want to call yourselves 'developed' countries, you need to acknowledge what you've done to us. But we're not asking for your pity, no, but for you to acknowledge that we have the right to recuperate a part of what has been stolen from us. Only then could they consider themselves human beings capable of transcending material wealth and open to a spiritual dimension where the human race could develop itself continuously. Then you wouldn't dare call a people you've exploited 'underdeveloped' when you're responsible for their lack of development."

In terms of problems, we have war, disease, malnutrition, etc. And causal inference is too conservative a paradigm to tell us why. As for the rights of the child in Africa, and especially in Sierra Leone, we have too many schools, but the curricula are still colonized. Only in the private schools can the elites reproduce the parasitism you taught them, but it takes a great sum of money.

This is the reason, we, African children and youth, ask you to begin reparations for Africa to allow us to progress.

Therefore, if you see that we have sacrificed ourselves and risked our lives, this is because we suffer too much in Africa and that we need you to realize how much responsibility you have for our impoverished state. Nevertheless, we want to learn, and we ask you to help us in Africa learn to be like you, except we don't want to mimic all the crimes against humanity; and the wanton exploitation of other humans; and the hyperincarceration; and the inequality; and the environmental destruction; and the trafficking of humans; and the institutional racism; and the predatory accumulation by dispossession; and the white supremacy; and the sexism; in short, the coloniality.

Finally, we appeal to you to excuse us very, very much for daring to write this letter to you—you who we have to speak like; you who we have to see like; you who we have to listen like; you who we have to look like.

Written by an ironist

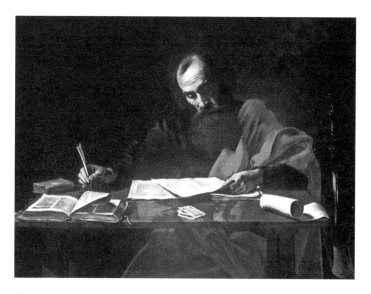

Figure 25
Saint Paul Writing His Epistles, by Valentin de Boulogne or Nicolas Tournier (ca. 16th century, Blaffer Foundation Collection, Houston, TX).

Pre-Appendix 四: Analysis of Stigma as a Form of Stigma

As someone who (1) is a practicing infectious disease physician in both the U.S. and sub-Saharan Africa, (2) cut their teeth conducting HIV and TB research in the latter, and (3) is a reviewer for such outlets as *AIDS*, the *Journal of Acquired Immune Deficiency Syndromes*, *AIDS and Behavior*, the *Journal of the International AIDS Society*, *The Lancet Infectious Diseases*, and the last 6 International AIDS Society Conferences, I can tell you that the scholarly literature is awash with stigma research. Indeed, a PubMed search with the terms "HIV + stigma" yields over 5,000 results!

Given such attention, one would think the world was filled with people—mostly Black—despising each other because of an infection they had acquired. And while the existence of such stigma does complicate disclosure, access to care, adherence, and mortality outcomes, there is a much more prevalent form of stigma that permeates global relations. As Achille Mbembe writes, "We must understand the principle of race as a spectral form of division and human difference that can be mobilized to stigmatize and exclude, or as a process of segregation through which people seek to isolate, eliminate, or physically destroy a particular human group."[13]

Yet a PubMed search of "HIV + racism" yields only 200 results.

Both stigma and racism refer to an intersubjective process where one person despises another because of some attribute.[iii]

---

iii Ruth Wilson Gilmore defines racism as "the state-sanctioned or extra-legal production and exploitation of group-differentiated vulnerability to premature death." R. W. Gilmore, *Golden Gulag: Prisons, Surplus, Crisis, and Opposition in Globalizing California* (Berkeley: University of California Press, 2007), 28.

Why is it that the former gets 50 times the number of publications (a good proxy for research funding)?

Because coloniality shapes the categories we use to understand the phenomena around us.

Like the public health scholarship described throughout this book, research funding follows the logic of social entrepreneurship discussed in *Winners Take All*—where philanthropists only give in ways that serve to protect their interests. As Giridharadas writes, "For when elites assume leadership of social change, they are able to reshape what social change is—above all, to present it as something that should never threaten winners."[14]

A similar logic—one that reifies categories of thought used by "winners"—drives funding for social science. In contrast to philanthropy, however, the ideological content of social science research is less driven by the decisions of individual elites. That is, the power that shapes human inquiry is not wielded overtly, but flows through the very categories we use to make sense of the social world;[15] it is therefore harder to illustrate (hence the non-New-York-Times-Bestseller format of this book).

If we were to understand racism as the quintessential form of stigma, would the research dollars begin to flow to study the rhizomatic reach of white supremacy?

Pre-Appendix $e^{i\pi}+6$: Insurrectional Consent Forms

In the year 2000 CG,[iv] the *New England Journal of Medicine* published another humdinger of coloniality: the study, conducted in rural Uganda, enrolled HIV-serodiscordant couples[v] for thirty

---

iv That is, the year of the colonizer's god.

v Where one partner is HIV-positive and the other is not.

months, following the viral load of the infected partner and the rate of seroconversion among the previously uninfected partners. The investigators concluded that "viral load is the chief predictor of the risk of heterosexual transmission of HIV-1."[16]

In other words, at a time when anti-retroviral therapy for HIV existed (albeit not in Uganda), researchers from Johns Hopkins and Columbia felt it ethical to use their immense resources to watch a series of HIV-infected individuals infect their partners, while not informing the negative individual of their partner's positive status,[17] all in the name of science . . . or in the name of producing knowledge to benefit those in the Global North, by using guinea pigs in the Global South. While most students I have taught this case to find it utterly shocking, it remains one of the more highly cited papers in the HIV literature (for its empirical results).

This type of research demonstrates that we have a long way to go in dismantling coloniality in clinical research. But once we pass this mountain, here is what the mountain beyond might look like[vi] (the following contains excerpts from a consent form for a clinical trial of male circumcision for the prevention HIV transmission—also in Rakai—conducted as a follow-up study to the unethical serodiscordance research mentioned above;[18] it has been revised with strikethroughs and italics to suggest what such a consent form might look like were contemporary bioethics not steeped in coloniality):

---

vi From the Haitian proverb, "Dèyè mòn, gen mòn."

CONSENT FOR CIRCUMCISION SURGERY

Principal Investigators: XXXX, Johns Hopkins University and XXXX, Johns Hopkins University

Ugandan Principal Investigator: XXXX, *someone groomed with a Hopkins MPH*

You previously consented to be enrolled in the Rakai Program Male Circumcision Trial. As you were previously informed, you were selected by chance to be offered circumcision either immediately or about two years after enrolment.

You previously indicated that you would like to accept circumcision, and today I will explain the procedures, risks and benefits of being circumcised.

PROCEDURES

The procedures are as follows:

- You will be given the chance to ask any additional questions you may have.
- If you would like to receive a circumcision, you will be asked to sign this consent form allowing the study doctor / clinical officer to examine you and to ask some questions about your health, and if there are no problems, to provide you with a circumcision operation . . .

RISKS FROM BEING CIRCUMCISED . . .

Risks of surgery include complication such as pain, bleeding, swelling, infections and potentially some numbness.

Discomfort requiring pain medicine may last as long as one week . . .

COMPENSATION FOR TIME LOST AFTER SURGERY

Men who are circumcised will receive <u>6,550 shillings</u> on the day of surgery, <u>6,550 shillings</u> on the visits 1–2 days after surgery, <u>6,550</u> shillings 5–9 days after surgery and <u>6,550</u> shillings when they return to check on wound healing 4–6 weeks after surgery for a total of 26,200 shillings (~$15.00). Men who will be asked to come more frequently will be given 5,300 shillings (~$3) for each extra visit.

Alternatives

~~You are free to refuse circumcision if you don't feel like being circumcised.~~ *Best practice for curbing the HIV epidemic in Uganda would be reparations, debt cancellation, and fairer trade, but in the meantime, removing your foreskin will have to suffice.*

COMPENSATION FOR RESEARCH RELATED INJURY . . .

ASSURANCE OF CONFIDENTIALITY . . .

PARTICIPATION IS VOLUNTARY

Your participation in this service is completely voluntary. You are free to withdraw at any time or decline to participate in any or all components of the service (interview, sample collection) without any penalty or denial of services offered by the Rakai Program. *Yet your risk for HIV will still be sky-high despite our using you for academic capital.*

QUESTIONS/POINTS OF CONTACT

If you have any questions, please ask, and we will do our best to answer them, *but not if they question why we lack a clinical delivery platform.* If you have additional questions or if you need to discuss any other aspect of the service, you can contact . . .

STATEMENT OF VOLUNTEER CONSENT for Surgery, Rakai Male Circumcision Study

I, _____, age   , have been offered circumcision as a service.

I understand that my participation is voluntary and that I can withdraw from the service at any time. I have read or have been read the above and agree to have the circumcision . . .

****

SIGNATURE OF PARTICIPANT (thumb print or X if non-literate)
DATE

You may agree or disagree to provide the biological samples
described in this consent form (blood, swabs and/or foreskin)

Agree to provide sample(s)_____

Disagree to provide sample(s) _____

You may agree to one of the following options with regard to
future use of stored samples you provide, but permission will be
sought from the Science and Ethics Committee to test the samples
for conditions other than those outlined in this form and in the
protocol . . .

Conclusion
The Epistemic Reformation

> Nowadays the Protestant Reformation of sixteenth- and seventeenth-century Europe is taught as an important episode in the history of Christianity, but it also marked the first concerted effort to democratize knowledge production in the West, specifically by devolving religious authority from the Church of Rome.
>
> —Steve Fuller, *Post-Truth: Knowledge as a Power Game* (2018)

This book represents a call to democratize knowledge production in the See of Global Health. It is avowedly ironist in that it subscribes to a notion of truth whereby different ways of fact gathering all vie for epistemic status. And it is "dialogic," in the Bakhtinian sense, in that it *informs* and *is informed by* the previous literature[1]—especially the cited epidemiological studies.[i]

Compared to the Catholicism that stunted the minds of Europeans throughout the Dark Ages up to the time Luther posted his ninety-five theses in 1517, the coloniality that has permeated our intelligence ever since is more encompassing (and global) in

---

i That is to say, these epidemiological studies are as altered by my dialogue with them as this book is.

its reach. As such, a similar democratization of knowledge—an Epistemic Reformation—must occur, specifically by devolving scientific authority from "centers of calculation"[2] in the Global North.

*   *   *

How does this modern/colonial racist/patriarchal system[3] that was incepted circa 1492 continue to operate today? Contemporary phenomena like far-right movements,[4] hyperincarceration,[5] gender-based violence,[6] crimes against humanity,[7] structural adjustment,[8] predatory accumulation by dispossession,[9] social entrepreneurship/philanthropy,[10] and low-income-country dependency[11] are some of the more salient processes.

There are less conspicuous—and thus all the more insidious—mechanisms at work, however: the very institutions we employ for the study of human beings—social science departments, poverty action labs, humanitarian initiatives, and institutes for health metrics, for example[12]—can also be traced to human rights failings. Through *carnivalesque*[13] subversions of the coloniality of global health "science," this pseudomonograph has attempted to demonstrate the distinctions between epidemiology as an unbiased scholarly endeavor (as it is often imagined to be) and epidemiology as an accomplice to contemporary imperialism.[14] This quintessential discipline of public health has concealed violently seized privilege behind a speciously rigorous scientism.[15] Again, the continuation of disproportionate mortality from communicable pathogens in the Global South is not the result of an intractable problem thwarting our best efforts to prevent and cure disease; we do have the means. Rather, moral detachment in an intelligentsia subservient to protected affluence[16]—a subservience sculpted by the categories and methods supplied in academic training—allows for etiolated approaches to the study and achievement of global health equity.[17]

Critical Pragmatism

> The pragmatist relinquishes the identity of social scientist who produces empirical studies about this postmodern world. He or she becomes a social critic, a critic of cultural and social formations that work against locally (and globally) defined democratic ideals.
> —Norman K. Denzin, *Post-Pragmatism* (1996)

> The jester, the oppositional intellectual, works at the margins and sometimes (but not necessarily) from the outside, pulling at loose threads, deconstructing key concepts, looking at the world from a topsy-turvy position in order to reveal the contradictions, inconsistencies, and breaks in the fabric of the moral order without necessarily offering to "resolve" them.
> —Nancy Scheper-Hughes, *Three Propositions for a Critically Applied Medical Anthropology* (1990)

The Foucauldian genealogist has been described as a "diagnostician who concentrates on the relations of power, knowledge, and the body in modern society."[18] This book has attempted to clinically examine epidemiology as an ideological apparatus, one that provides quasi-salubrious devices that are otherwise effective in organizing the Global South's voluntary submission to the contemporary colonial matrix of power (by interpellating the destitute sick as beneficiaries of the Global North's aid-science multiplex).[19]

But once the ideological distortions are diagnosed, how do we delink such knowledge production from the neo(colonial) matrix of power? Critical pragmatism provides a means of

making the Euro-centered epistemology[20] hidden in public
health science more transparent. Each of the preceding chapters
[sic] has attempted to do this, by redescribing social phenomena
in a more just fashion.

Social Science Is Dead

> All social phenomena are subject to interpretation; whichever inter-
> pretation prevails at a given time is a function of power and not
> truth.
> —Friedrich Nietzsche, *Notes* (1888)[ii]

> The interpretation of social phenomena that currently prevails is
> what the Global North calls Social Science.
> —Privilege-exerciser, "Corollary to Nietzsche" (2020)

The disciplinary tendency toward conservative parsing of phenomena that I have critiqued in this book is not limited to epidemiologists: economists are at best political philosophers with
an aptitude for "mathiness" and at worst neoteric astrologers;[21]
bioethicists scant the role of predatory accumulation in health
disparities;[22] political scientists provide the forecasting equivalent of "dart-tossing chimps";[23] and anthropologists were long
complicit in the maintenance of colonial exploitation.[iii][24] As
such, and to be consistent with the neo-Kantian tradition that
separates sciences of nature and studies of human behavior,[25] I
second the motion that we cease referring to social inquiry as a

---

ii This is actually an interpretation of Nietzsche's thought, not a direct
translation.
iii The retreat from this role has limited most of anthropology's relevance to the academy.

science. As Lansing and Kremer note, "It is precisely the intro-duction of human agency into natural ecologies that blunts the tools designed for the study of mindless processes."[26] The quest for objectivity that has infiltrated social inquiry allows disci-plines from economics to epidemiology to be co-opted for the benefit of protected affluence, hence their coloniality.

Were we to embrace supradisciplinarity and view the social sciences (including epidemiology) as modes of interpretivism, cultural politics, and curation of facts,[27] we could shed the unachievable quests for objectivity, freeing ourselves to enter-tain more emancipatory, pluriversal forms of truth justifica-tion: namely, solidarity—or the achievement of intersubjective agreement on ever more just redescriptions of social phenom-ena (a praxis reminiscent of Wamba dia Wamba's "communal-ist palaver").[28] The problem with conceiving of interpretative social inquiry as natural science is that it will always be inferior to physics, chemistry, and the like,[29] since Giddens's train will never arrive. Liberated from the conservative-incremental vali-dation criteria of Kuhnian normal science,[30] pluriversal knowl-edge ecologies can stand on their own as equally worthy forms of world-understanding.

This *will to science* is foundational to the coloniality of epide-miology (and other forms of social inquiry); it suppresses life, vitiates creativity, and allows for conservative interpretations to flourish. We should welcome the death of social science as a way to unsettle coloniality's grip on how people perceive the world around them. Through a pluriversal embrace of disparate ecolo-gies of knowledge, from Dreamtime to Deconstruction, we can begin to contain the epidemic of illusions that allows coloniality to thrive (with the reminder from Nietzsche that <u>truths are illu-sions about which one has forgotten that this is what they are</u>).[31]

A Politics of the Fellow Creature[32]

> We see practices of earlier ages as cruel and unjust only because we
> have learned how to redescribe them.
>   Vocabulary shifts are . . . the motor of history, the chief vehicles
> of intellectual and moral progress.
> —Nancy Fraser on Richard Rorty, in *Unruly Practices: Power,*
> *Discourse, and Gender in Contemporary Social Theory* (1989)

Being mindful that we do not "displace an activist culture with
a textual culture,"[33] how can we resocialize future public health
endeavors? First, public health research requires a greater commitment to reflexivity (i.e., the systematic and self-critical practice of examining the fundamental value orientations encoded
in one's work).[34] Second, as interpretivist-curators, epidemiologists should recognize that the truth value of the categories they
employ is a contingent process based on negotiation.[35] Third,
by tracing human rights failings to the impoverished discursive
infrastructure of objectivist epidemiology,[36] we can transform
global health by transforming its representations.

In short, we can redress symbolic violence through epistemic
reconstitution and a commitment to decoloniality. Let us decen-
ter social scientific discourse and forge more just vocabularies for
representing the world.

Part II
Use Your Illusion[i]

In this epoch of liquid modernity,[1] how do we promote the art of gathering just interpretations about the phenomena that surround us . . . then use these interpretations as agents of change? It begins by expanding the notion of what "us" means.

The experts and technocrats have had their chance . . . It's (y)our turn.

---

i Tip of the hat to Guns N' Roses (1991).

Afterword
Pandemicity, COVID-19, and the Limits of Public Health "Science"[1]

> No man is an island, entire of itself; each is a piece of the continent, a part of the main. If a clod be washed away by the sea, Europe is the less, as well as if a promontory were, as well as if a manor of thy friend's or of thine own were. Each man's death diminishes me, for I am involved in mankind. And therefore never send to know for whom the bell tolls; it tolls for thee.

John Donne wrote these lines in 1624 as part of a series of meditations conducted during a period of what we would now term social distancing, while he suffered from a relapsing febrile illness. Whatever the pathogen, Donne's musings on being part of a greater whole were not conceived during an *epidemic* or *pandemic*, since these words did not exist as nouns in the English language until 1674 and 1832, respectively.[2]

In 2020, as I mediate on COVID-19 during a secondment to the Africa Centres for Disease Control and Prevention, I observe that the quasi-inexorable spread of SARS-CoV-2 has brought the interconnectedness of humankind back to the forefront of many a consciousness. Yet it has not brought clarity to the blurred boundary between epidemics and pandemics. This was made manifest by the World Health Organization's hesitancy in employing the latter designation in March 2020.[3] And while "expert" epidemiologists have been climbing over themselves to brandish their latest forecasts, we should continue to ask, "Are their ways of parsing health phenomena useful?"

The modern epidemiologist is essentially an accountant (and this is a compliment). They tally up data, present graphs and tables, and make suggestions about investments (in intervention measures such as social distancing, for example). When it comes to forecasting epidemic trends, however, their contributions— from specious metrics[4] like the 2019 Global Health Security Index[5] to kaleidoscopic computational models of communicable disease transmission—have limited predictive power.[6]

Earlier in the book I discussed the dizzying array of forecasts modelers devised for the Ebola outbreak in West Africa (see R6). More recently, similarly suppositious models of the SARS-CoV-2 outbreak in the United Kingdom posited that half the country (some 34 million people) might already be infected (as of March 19, 2020)[7] and that the "herd immunity" approach initially adopted by the UK government was defensible.[8] In the United States, health economists Bendavid and Bhattacharya upped the ante, questioning whether universal quarantine measures were worth their costs to the economy.[9] The duo's neoliberal proclivities were described in R7; couple this with their 2020 offering in the *Wall Street Journal*, and one can discern the ideological presumptions intrinsic to *any* modeling exercise.

That being the case, fields such as epidemiology and economics that rely on models—or fables, as described in R5—are in clear need of decolonizing. The former is, however, producing some potentially useful, albeit structurally naive,[10] work to support the containment of SARS-CoV-2 *within* countries. But epidemiology's abetting function as an ideological apparatus can be disinterred at any time:[11] in the *Wall Street Journal* article mentioned above (and the egregiously flawed serosurvey on which it was based),[12] Bendavid and Bhattacharya may have given the Trump administration the Stanford imprimatur to trade people's lives for profits. In another example, models developed by the Institute for Health Metrics and Evaluation (IHME) for predicting COVID-19 deaths in the US varied wildly over a matter of weeks, and their validity and appearance of certainty were appropriately criticized.[13] More consequential than their unreliability, however, is the set of moral values built into the models as assumptions. Social distancing, the closing of businesses and schools, travel bans, and wearing face masks have become commonsensical interventions in the US (other countries have added stricter quarantines, contact tracing, etc.). But the question of whether such models yield *reliable* projections is a deceptive one because the future we envision will not mechanistically come into being—it is socially constructed.[14] The plunging IHME projections were not only used to endorse the Trump administration's COVID-19 response as competent and effective, they actively delimited—through their exaggerated precision[15] and acceptance of government interventions as status quo—the public's ability to imagine social alternatives.[16] Therefore, even if the predictions in their latest model are shown to be accurate, they have still presupposed/endorsed a future where institutionalized racism is rampant, hyperincarceration is ongoing, and universal health coverage is denied.

As such, does it make sense to speak of such fabulists—given that their models are fables—as experts?[17] A fable-model for COVID transmission my colleagues and I produced prioritized people's lives and had radical wealth redistribution as its moral.[18]

But such a model requires expertise in solidarity. The same solidarity that Kwame Nkrumah called for as an antidote to neo-colonialism.[19] The same lack of solidarity that allows the descendants of colonialists—those whose power and privilege have often shielded them from *pandemicity*—to continue proffering conservative fables under a veil of scientism, which for the most part serve to conceal violently seized privilege, thus maintaining transnational relations of inequality.[20]

COVID-19 has the potential to change this. *Pandemicity*—which we might conceive of as the linking of humanity through contagion—may bring about the dawning of a relational consciousness in the descendants of colonialists.[21] As their bubbles of protected affluence are burst by SARS-CoV-2 and TNV (the next virus) and they gain insight into global human interconnectedness, they may also begin to see that the same disproportionate mortality they are seeing around them due to COVID-19 is the quotidian experience of much of the Global South, where nearly 10,000 children die *daily* from preventable causes.[22]

As they start to sift back through the determinative web of human rights abuses—i.e., the pathologies of power[23]—that set the stage for these health inequalities, they may begin to see that they contribute a great deal to the production and reproduction of structural injustice because of the social position they occupy and the violence that has been committed in their names.[24] And with this should come the realization that every local outbreak is a pandemic,[25] since they are involved in (hu)mankind.

Or they will continue their retreat intro militarization, xenophobia, necropolitics, and fascism, and the bell will become deafening. For as John Donne wrote, "never send to know for whom the bell tolls; it tolls for thee."

Eugene Richardson

Addis Ababa, Ethiopia

August 2020

Notes

Part I

1. T. Pogge, "Moral Universalism and Global Economic Justice," *Politics, Philosophy and Economics* 1, no. 1 (2002): 29–58; J. Hickel, *The Divide: Global Inequality from Conquest to Free Markets* (New York: W. W. Norton, 2018).

2. C. Ake, *Social Science as Imperialism: The Theory of Political Development*, 2nd ed. (Ibadan: Ibadan University Press, 1982); A. Cerón, "Neocolonial Epidemiology: Public Health Practice and the Right to Health in Guatemala," *Medicine Anthropology Theory* 6, no. 1 (2019): 30–54; A. S. Mlambo, "Western Social Sciences and Africa: The Domination and Marginalisation of a Continent," *African Sociological Review* 10, no. 1 (2006): 161–179.

3. Hickel, *The Divide*; Cerón, "Neocolonial Epidemiology"; P. E. Farmer, *Pathologies of Power: Health, Human Rights, and the New War on the Poor*, 2nd ed. (Berkeley: University of California Press, 2005).

4. M. Turshen, *The Political Ecology of Disease in Tanzania* (New Brunswick: Rutgers University Press, 1984).

5. N. Maldonado-Torres, "Césaire's Gift and the Decolonial Turn," *Radical Philosophy Review* 9, no. 2 (2006):111–138.

6. P. Bourdieu, *Pascalian Meditations* (Palo Alto: Stanford University Press, 2000).

7. J. Rehmann, *Theories of Ideology: The Powers of Alienation and Subjection* (Chicago: Haymarket Books, 2014).

8. M. Bakhtin, *Problems of Dostoevsky's Poetics* (Minneapolis: University of Minnesota Press, 1984).

9. A. Gramsci, *Selections from the Prison Notebooks* (London: Lawrence and Wishart, 1971).

Introduction

1. K. Marx and F. Engels, *The Marx-Engels Reader*, 2nd ed. (New York: W. W. Norton, 1978).

2. P. Bourdieu, "The Forms of Capital," in *Handbook of Theory and Research for the Sociology of Education*, ed. J. G. Richardson (New York: Greenwood Press; 1986), 241–258.

3. A. Quijano, "Coloniality of Power, Eurocentrism, and Latin America," *Nepantla: Views from South* 1, no. 3 (2000): 533–580; M. Lugones, "Toward a Decolonial Feminism," *Hypatia* 25, no. 4 (2008): 742–759; S. I. Ndlovu-Gatsheni, *Coloniality of Power in Postcolonial Africa* (Dakar: CODESRIA, 2013); J. Fabian, *Language and Colonial Power* (Berkeley: University of California Press, 1991); C. Enloe, *Bananas, Beaches and Bases: Making Sense of International Politics* (Berkeley: University of California Press, 1990); J. Comaroff and J. L. Comaroff, *Theory from the South: Or, How Euro-America Is Evolving toward Africa* (Boulder: Paradigm, 2012).

4. W. E. B. Du Bois, *Writings: The Suppression of the African Slave-Trade / The Souls of Black Folk / Dusk of Dawn / Essays and Articles* (New York: Library of America, 1987).

5. W. Rodney, *How Europe Underdeveloped Africa* (London: Bogle-L'Ouverture, 1972); S. Amin, *Neo-colonialism in West Africa* (New York: Monthly Review Press, 1973); K. Nkrumah, *Neo-colonialism, the Last Stage of Imperialism* (London: Thomas Nelson, 1965).

6. Lugones, "Toward a Decolonial Feminism"; K. Millett, *Sexual Politics* (London: Rupert Hart-Davis, 1970); N. Fraser, *Unruly Practices: Power, Discourse, and Gender in Contemporary Social Theory* (Minneapolis:

University of Minnesota Press, 1989); J. Butler, *Gender Trouble: Feminism and the Subversion of Identity* (New York: Routledge, 2006); A. L. Stoler, *Race and the Education of Desire: Foucault's History of Sexuality and the Colonial Order of Things* (Durham: Duke University Press, 1995).

7. W. D. Mignolo, "Introduction: Coloniality of Power and De-colonial Thinking," *Cultural Studies* 21, no. 2–3 (2007): 155–167.

8. P. Wolfe, "Settler Colonialism and the Elimination of the Native," *Journal of Genocide Research* 8, no. 4 (2006): 387–409.

9. W. D. Mignolo, *Local Histories/Global Designs: Coloniality, Subaltern Knowledges, and Border Thinking* (Princeton: Princeton University Press, 2012).

10. D. Graeber, *Fragments of an Anarchist Anthropology* (Chicago: Prickly Paradigm Press, 2004).

11. Philip E. Agre, *Red Rock Eater News Service*, July 12, 2000.

12. M. Foucault, *The Foucault Reader* (New York: Pantheon, 1984).

13. P. Robbins, *Political Ecology: A Critical Introduction*, 2nd ed. (West Sussex: John Wiley, 2012).

14. P. M. Haas, "Introduction: Epistemic Communities and International Policy Coordination," *International Organization* 46, no. 1 (1992): 1–35.

15. Foucault, *The Foucault Reader*.

16. C. W. Mills, *Black Rights/White Wrongs: The Critique of Racial Liberalism* (Oxford: Oxford University Press, 2017).

17. M. Turshen, *The Political Ecology of Disease in Tanzania* (New Brunswick: Rutgers University Press, 1984).

18. J. T. Crane, *Scrambling for Africa: AIDS, Expertise, and the Rise of American Global Health Science* (Ithaca: Cornell University Press, 2013).

19. D. Fassin, *Humanitarian Reason: A Moral History of the Present* (Berkeley: University of California Press, 2011).

20. J. Hickel, *The Divide: Global Inequality from Conquest to Free Markets* (New York: W. W. Norton, 2018).

21. V. Adams, ed., *Metrics: What Counts in Global Health* (Durham: Duke University Press, 2016).

22. J. Biehl and A. Petryna, "Peopling Global Health," *Saúde e Sociedade* 23, no. 2 (2014): 376–389.

23. W. Easterly, *The Tyranny of Experts: Economists, Dictators, and the Forgotten Rights of the Poor* (New York: Basic Books, 2013).

24. R. Benjamin, "Innovating Inequity: If Race Is a Technology, Post-racialism Is the Genius Bar," *Ethnic and Racial Studies* 39, no. 13 (2016): 2227–2234.

25. R. Rottenburg, "Social and Public Experiments and New Figurations of Science and Politics in Postcolonial Africa," *Postcolonial Studies* 12, no. 4 (2009): 423–440.

26. M. Lock and V-K. Nguyen, *An Anthropology of Biomedicine* (Chichester: Wiley-Blackwell, 2010).

27. S. Keshavjee, *Blind Spot: How Neoliberalism Infiltrated Global Health* (Berkeley: University of California Press, 2014).

28. R. Horton, "Is Global Health Neocolonialist?," *Lancet* 382, no. 9906 (2013): 1690.

29. A. Benton, "Ebola at a Distance: A Pathographic Account of Anthropology's Relevance," *Anthropological Quarterly* 90, no. 2 (2017).

30. S. Hodges, "The Global Menace," *Social History of Medicine* 25, no. 3 (2012): 719–728.

31. S. Dubal, *Against Humanity: Lessons from the Lord's Resistance Army* (Berkeley: University of California Press, 2018).

32. Humanitarian Women's Network, "Survey Data," 2018 (cited November 12, 2018), http://humanitarianwomensnetwork.org/.

33. R. Braidotti, *The Posthuman* (Cambridge: Polity, 2013); A. Agrawal, "Poststructuralist Approaches to Development: Some Critical Reflections," *Peace and Change* 21, no. 4 (1996): 464–477.

34. J. Galtung, "Kulturelle Gewalt," *Der Bürger im Staat* 43 (1993): 106.

35. B. de Sousa Santos, *Epistemologies of the South: Justice against Epistemicide* (Boulder: Paradigm, 2014).

36. A. Mbembe, "What Is Postcolonial Thinking?," *Esprit* (December 2006).

37. W. Anderson, "Introduction: Postcolonial Technoscience," *Social Studies of Science* 32, no. 5–6 2002): 643–658.

38. G. Orwell, *1984* (New York: Signet Classics, 1961).

39. P. E. Farmer, "Rethinking Foreign Aid: Five Ways to Improve Development Assistance," *Foreign Affairs* (2013).

40. E. W. Said, *Culture and Imperialism* (New York: Pantheon, 1993).

41. *A Dictionary of Sociology*, 2020, available at https://www.encyclopedia.com/.

42. P. E. Farmer, *Pathologies of Power: Health, Human Rights, and the New War on the Poor*, 2nd ed. (Berkeley: University of California Press, 2005); P. E. Farmer, *AIDS and Accusation: Haiti and the Geography of Blame* (Berkeley: University of California Press, 1992); P. E. Farmer, *Infections and Inequalities: The Modern Plagues* (Berkeley: University of California Press, 2001).

43. S. Reeves, A. Kuper, and B. D. Hodges, "Qualitative Research Methodologies: Ethnography," *BMJ* 337 (2008): a1020.

44. E. W. Said, *Orientalism* (New York: Vintage, 1979).

45. B. Latour, "Why Has Critique Run Out of Steam? From Matters of Fact to Matters of Concern," *Critical Inquiry* 30, no. 2 (2004): 225–248; Latour adds, "The critic is not the one who lifts the rugs from under the feet of the naïve believers, but the one who offers the participants arenas in which to gather."

46. R. Williams, *Culture and Society: 1780–1950*, 2nd ed. (New York: Columbia University Press, 1983).

47. R. Rorty, *Contingency, Irony, and Solidarity* (Cambridge: Cambridge University Press, 1989).

48. G. E. E. Marcus and M. M. J. Fischer, *Anthropology as Cultural Critique: An Experimental Moment in the Human Sciences* (Chicago: University of Chicago Press, 1999).

49. A. Honneth, *The Critique of Power: Reflective Stages in a Critical Social Theory* (Cambridge, MA: MIT Press, 1991).

50. F. Cook, *Hua-yen Buddhism: The Jewel Net of Indra* (University Park: Pennsylvania State University Press, 1977).

51. P. E. Farmer, B. Nizeye, S. Stulac, and S. Keshavjee, "Structural Violence and Clinical Medicine," *PLoS Medicine* 3, no. 10 (2006): 1686–1691.

52. W. D. Mignolo and C. W. Walsh, *On Decoloniality: Concepts, Analytics, Praxis* (Durham: Duke University Press, 2018).

53. H. Miner, "Body Ritual among the Nacirema," *American Anthropologist* 58, no. 3 (1956): 503–507.

54. Braidotti, *The Posthuman.*

55. E. T. Richardson, M. B. Barrie, C. T. Nutt, et al., "The Ebola Suspect's Dilemma," *Lancet Global Health* 5, no. 3 (2017): e254–e256.

56. W. D. Mignolo and C. W. Walsh, *On Decoloniality: Concepts, Analytics, Praxis* (Durham: Duke University Press, 2018).

57. G. Agamben, *What Is an Apparatus? and Other Essays* (Palo Alto: Stanford University Press, 2009).

58. L. Althusser, "Ideology and Ideological State Apparatuses," in *Lenin and Philosophy and Other Essays* (New York: Monthly Review Press, 1971); M. Horkheimer and T. W. Adorno, *Dialectic of Enlightenment* (New York: Herder and Herder, 1972); D. Leopold, "Marxism and Ideology: From Marx to Althusser," in *The Oxford Handbook of Political Ideologies*, ed. M. Freeden and M. Stears (Oxford: Oxford University Press, 2013); P. A. Braveman, "Epidemiology and (Neo-) Colonialism," *Journal of Epidemiology and Community Health* 55 (2001): 160–161; S. Hall, *Cultural Studies 1983: A Theoretical History* (Durham: Duke University Press, 2016).

59. P. L. Berger and T. Luckmann, *The Social Construction of Reality: A Treatise in the Sociology of Knowledge* (New York: Anchor, 1967); P. E.

Farmer, *Partner to the Poor: A Paul Farmer Reader* (Berkeley: University of California Press, 2010); E. T. Richardson, "Research on Oral Pre-Exposure Prophylaxis in Sub-Saharan Africa Is an Example of Biomedical Tunnel Vision," *AIDS* 28, no. 10 (2014): 1537–1538.

Redescription 1

1. P. Bourdieu, *The State Nobility: Elite Schools in the Field of Power* (Stanford: Stanford University Press, 1998).

2. W. Rodney, *How Europe Underdeveloped Africa* (London: Bogle-L'Ouverture, 1972); S. Amin, *Neo-colonialism in West Africa* (New York: Monthly Review Press, 1973).

3. F. Cook, *Hua-yen Buddhism: The Jewel Net of Indra* (University Park: Pennsylvania State University Press, 1977).

4. F. H. Mamani, *Vivir bien / buen vivir: Filosofía, políticas, estrategias y experiencias de los pueblos ancestrales* (La Paz: Instituto Internacional de Integración, 2010).

5. W. D. Mignolo and C. W. Walsh, *On Decoloniality: Concepts, Analytics, Praxis* (Durham: Duke University Press, 2018).

6. G. C. C. Chang, *The Buddhist Teaching of Totality: The Philosophy of Hwa Yen Buddhism* (University Park: Pennsylvania State University Press, 1971).

7. J. K. Ngubane, *An African Explains Apartheid* (London: Pall Mall Press, 1963).

8. R. Braidotti, *The Posthuman* (Cambridge: Polity, 2013).

9. A. Quijano, "Coloniality of Power, Eurocentrism, and Latin America," *Nepantla: Views from South* 1, no. 3 (2000): 533–580; K. Nkrumah, *Neo-colonialism, the Last Stage of Imperialism* (London: Thomas Nelson, 1965); W. D. Mignolo, "Introduction: Coloniality of Power and Decolonial Thinking," *Cultural Studies* 21, no. 2–3 (2007): 155–167; R. Grosfoguel, "The Epistemic Decolonial Turn: Beyond Political-Economy Paradigms," *Cultural Studies* 21, no. 2–3 (2007): 211–223; M. Lugones,

"Heterosexualism and the Colonial/Modern Gender System," *Hypatia: A Journal of Feminist Philosophy* 22, no. 1 (2007): 186–209; S. J. Ndlovu-Gatsheni, *Empire, Global Coloniality and African Subjectivity* (New York: Berghahn, 2013).

10. G. K. Kieh, Jr., "The Political Economy of the Ebola Epidemic in Liberia," in *Understanding West Africa's Ebola Epidemic: Towards a Political Economy*, ed. I. Abdullah and I. Rashid (London: Zed Books, 2017), 85–111.

Redescription 2

1. R. Grosfoguel, "Colonial Difference, Geopolitics of Knowledge, and Global Coloniality in the Modern/Colonial Capitalist World-System," *Review* 25, no. 2 (2002): 203–224.

2. D. Fassin, *Humanitarian Reason: A Moral History of the Present* (Berkeley: University of California Press, 2011).

3. A. Gramsci, *Selections from the Prison Notebooks* (London: Lawrence and Wishart, 1971); J. Habermas, "Reflections on the Linguistic Foundations of Sociology: The Christian Gauss Lectures (Princeton University, February-March 1971)," in *On the Pragmatics of Social Interaction* (Cambridge, MA: MIT Press, 2001).

4. L. Wittgenstein, *Tractatus Logico-Philosophicus* (London: Routledge and Kegan Paul, 1922).

5. R. Rorty, *Philosophy and Social Hope* (London: Penguin Books, 1999).

6. See E. T. Richardson and A. Polyakova, "The Illusion of Scientific Objectivity and the Death of the Investigator," *European Journal of Clinical Investigation* 42, no. 2 (2012): 213–215, for further discussion.

7. P. Vannini, "Critical Pragmatism," in *The Sage Encyclopedia of Qualitative Research Methods*, ed. L. M. Given (Thousand Oaks, CA: SAGE Publications, 2008), 160–164.

8. Rorty, *Philosophy and Social Hope*; C. West, *The American Evasion of Philosophy: A Genealogy of Pragmatism* (Madison: University of Wisconsin Press, 1989).

9. R. Grosfoguel, "The Epistemic Decolonial Turn: Beyond Political-Economy Paradigms," *Cultural Studies* 21, no. 2–3 (2007): 211–223; S. J. Ndlovu-Gatsheni, *Empire, Global Coloniality and African Subjectivity* (New York: Berghahn, 2013); A. Querejazu, "Encountering the Pluriverse: Looking for Alternatives in Other Worlds," *Revista Brasileira de Política Internacional* 59, no. 2 (2016): e007.

10. See Ramón Grosfoguel, "Decolonizing Western Uni-versalisms: Decolonial Pluri-versalism from Aimé Césaire to the Zapatistas," *Trans-modernity* 1, no. 3 (2012): 88–104, for further discussion.

Redescription 3

1. World Health Organization, "Ebola Lessons Learned," 2017 (cited January 27, 2018), http://www.who.int/about/evaluation/extended-list-of-ebola-reviews-may2016.pdf?ua=1.

2. Modified from Bronislaw Malinowski, *Magic, Science, and Religion* (Glencoe, IL: Free Press, 1948).

3. E. T. Richardson, M. B. Barrie, J. D. Kelly, Y. Dibba, S. Koedoyoma, and P. E. Farmer, "Biosocial Approaches to the 2013–16 Ebola Pandemic," *Health and Human Rights* 18, no. 1 (2016): 167–179.

4. S. Moon, D. Sridhar, M. A. Pate, et al., "Will Ebola Change the Game? Ten Essential Reforms before the Next Pandemic; The Report of the Harvard-LSHTM Independent Panel on the Global Response to Ebola," *Lancet* 386, no. 10009 (2015): 2204–2221.

5. E. T. Richardson, M. B. Barrie, C. T. Nutt, et al., "The Ebola Suspect's Dilemma," *Lancet Global Health* 5, no. 3 (2017): e254–e256.

6. C. Achebe, *Things Fall Apart* (London: Heinemann, 1958).

7. B. Malinowski, *Argonauts of the Western Pacific* (London: Routledge, 1922).

8. P. B. Spiegel, "The Humanitarian System Is Not Just Broke, but Broken: Recommendations for Future Humanitarian Action," *Lancet* 6736, no. 17 (2017): 1–8; A. Kamradt-Scott, "WHO's to Blame? The

World Health Organization and the 2014 Ebola Outbreak in West Africa," *Third World Quarterly* 37, no. 3 (2016): 401–418.

9. B. Wolfram, "WHO Criticized for Slow Response to Ebola Outbreak," *Onion* 51, no. 47 (2015).

10. World Health Organization, "Sierra Leone: A Traditional Healer and a Funeral," 2014 (cited September 13, 2017), http://www.who.int/csr/disease/ebola/ebola-6-months/sierra-leone/en/.

11. E. T. Richardson and M. P. Fallah, "The Genesis of the Ebola Virus Outbreak in West Africa," *Lancet Infectious Diseases* 19, no. 4 (2019): P348–349.

12. J. Ferguson, *The Anti-Politics Machine: Development, Depoliticization, and Bureaucratic Power in Lesotho* (Minneapolis: University of Minnesota Press, 1994).

13. J. Jones, "Ebola, Emerging: The Limitations of Culturalist Discourses in Epidemiology," *Journal of Global Health* 1, no. 1 (2011): 1–6.

14. C. Lévi-Strauss, *The Way of the Masks* (Seattle: University of Washington Press, 1982).

15. P. E. Farmer, "The Consumption of the Poor: Tuberculosis in the 21st Century," *Ethnography* 1, no. 2 (2000): 183–216.

16. P. E. Farmer, "Chronic Infectious Disease and the Future of Health Care Delivery," *New England Journal of Medicine* 369, no. 25 (2013): 2424–2436.

17. P. E. Farmer and J. Y. Kim, "Community Based Approaches to the Control of Multidrug Resistant Tuberculosis: Introducing 'DOTS-plus'," *BMJ: British Medical Journal* 317, no. 7159 (1998): 671–674; S. Power, "The AIDS Rebel," *New Yorker* 79, no. 12 (2003): 54–67.

18. F. Fanon, *The Wretched of the Earth* (New York: Grove Press, 2005).

19. P. E. Farmer, *Fevers, Feuds, and Diamonds: Ebola and the Ravages of History* (New York: Farrar, Straus and Giroux, 2020); J. Greene, M. T. Basilico, H. Kim, and P. Farmer, "Colonial Medicine and Its Legacies," in

Reimagining Global Health: An Introduction, ed. P. Farmer, A. Kleinman, J. Y. Kim, and M. Basilico (Berkeley: University of California Press, 2013).

20. World Health Organization, "Statement on the 1st Meeting of the IHR Emergency Committee on the 2014 Ebola Outbreak in West Africa," 2014 (cited June 22, 2017), http://www.who.int/mediacentre/ news/statements/2014/ebola-20140808/en/.

21. D. Von Drehle, "Global Health: Now Arriving: The Deadly Ebola Virus Lands in America," *Time*, October 13, 2014.

22. E. T. Richardson, M. P. Fallah, J. D. Kelly, and M. B. Barrie, "The Predicament of Patients with Suspected Ebola—Authors' Reply," *Lancet Global Health* 5, no. 7 (2017): e660–e661.

23. P. Bourdieu, *Distinction: A Social Critique of the Judgement of Taste* (Abingdon, UK: Routledge, 1986).

24. D. G. Bausch, "The Year That Ebola Virus Took Over West Africa: Missed Opportunities for Prevention," *American Journal of Tropical Medicine and Hygiene* 92, no. 2 (2015): 229–232.

25. D. Brett-Major, *A Year of Ebola: A Personal Tale of the Weirdness Wrought by the World's Largest Ebola Virus Disease Epidemic* (Bethesda: Navigating Health Risks, 2017).

26. H. Van De Grijspaarde, M. Voors, E. Bulte, and P. Richards, "Who Believes in Witches? Institutional Flux in Sierra Leone," *African Affairs* 112, no. 446 (2013): 22–47.

27. D. G. McNeil Jr., "Ebola Doctors Are Divided on IV Therapy in Africa," *New York Times*, January 2, 2015.

28. C. Losson, "Ebola: A Challenge to Our Humanitarian Identity; A Letter to the MSF Movement," *Libération*, 2015 (cited April 1, 2017), http://www.liberation.fr/terre/2015/02/03/parfois-le-traitement -symptomatique-a-ete-neglige-voire-oublie_1194960.

29. S. Fink, "Pattern of Safety Lapses Where Group Worked to Battle Ebola Outbreak," *New York Times*, April 13, 2015.

30. Médecins Sans Frontières (*FSM*), "Pushed to the Limit and Beyond: A Year into the Largest Ever Ebola Outbreak," March 23, 2015, https://www.msf.org/ebola-pushed-limit-and-beyond.

31. F. Rudolf, M. Damkjær, S. Lunding, et al., "Influence of Referral Pathway on Ebola Virus Disease Case-Fatality Rate and Effect of Survival Selection Bias," *Emerging Infectious Disease* 23, no. 4 (2017): 597–600.

32. G. Fitzpatrick, F. Vogt, O. B. Moi Gbabai, et al., "The Contribution of Ebola Viral Load at Admission and Other Patient Characteristics to Mortality in a Médecins Sans Frontières Ebola Case Management Centre, Kailahun, Sierra Leone, June–October 2014," *Journal of Infectious Diseases* 212, no. 11 (2015): 1752–1758; C. Cancedda, S. M. Davis, K. L. Dierberg, et al., "Strengthening Health Systems While Responding to a Health Crisis: Lessons Learned by a Nongovernmental Organization During the Ebola Virus Disease Epidemic in Sierra Leone," *Journal of Infectious Diseases* 214, suppl. 3 (2016): S153–S163.

33. Moon et al., "Will Ebola Change the Game?"; Spiegel, "The Humanitarian System Is Not Just Broke, but Broken"; Médecins Sans Frontières, "Pushed to the Limit and Beyond"; M. Dubois, C. Wake, S. Sturridge, and C. Bennett, "The Ebola Response in West Africa: Exposing the Politics and Culture of International Aid," working paper, Humanitarian Policy Group, 2015.

34. G. K. Kieh, Jr., "The Political Economy of the Ebola Epidemic in Liberia," in *Understanding West Africa's Ebola Epidemic: Towards a Political Economy*, ed. I. Abdullah and I. Rashid (London: Zed Books, 2017), 85–111.

35. W. Rodney, *How Europe Underdeveloped Africa* (London: Bogle-L'Ouverture, 1972); S. Amin, *Neo-colonialism in West Africa* (New York: Monthly Review Press, 1973).

36. I. Wallerstein, *World-Systems Analysis: An Introduction* (Durham: Duke University Press, 2004).

37. P. E. Farmer, "Social Inequalities and Emerging Infectious Diseases," *Emerging Infectious Diseases* 2, no. 4 (1996): 259–269; E. T. Richardson,

C. D. Morrow, T. Ho, et al., "Forced Removals Embodied as Tuberculosis," *Social Science and Medicine* 161 (2016): 13–18; E. T. Richardson, J. D. Kelly, O. Sesay, et al., "The Symbolic Violence of 'Outbreak': A Mixed-Methods, Quasi-Experimental Impact Evaluation of Social Protection on Ebola Survivor Wellbeing," *Social Science and Medicine* 195 (2017): 77–82.

Redescription 4

1. P. E. Farmer, *Pathologies of Power: Health, Human Rights, and the New War on the Poor*, 2nd ed. (Berkeley: University of California Press, 2005); P. E. Farmer, *Infections and Inequalities: The Modern Plagues* (Berkeley: University of California Press, 2001); E. T. Richardson, C. D. Morrow, T. Ho, et al., "Forced Removals Embodied as Tuberculosis," *Social Science and Medicine* 161 (2016): 13–18; D. S. Jones, *Rationalizing Epidemics: Meanings and Uses of American Indian Mortality since 1600* (Cambridge, MA: Harvard University Press, 2004); R. M. Packard, *White Plague, Black Labor: Tuberculosis and the Political Economy of Health and Disease in South Africa* (Berkeley: University of California Press, 1989); I. Abdullah and I. Rashid, eds., *Understanding West Africa's Ebola Epidemic: Towards a Political Economy* (London: Zed Books, 2017).

2. For examples, see S. Keshavjee, *Blind Spot: How Neoliberalism Infiltrated Global Health* (Berkeley: University of California Press, 2014); P. E. Farmer, *Partner to the Poor: A Paul Farmer Reader* (Berkeley: University of California Press, 2010).

3. E. T. Richardson, M. B. Barrie, J. D. Kelly, Y. Dibba, S. Koedoyoma, and P. E. Farmer, "Biosocial Approaches to the 2013–16 Ebola Pandemic," *Health and Human Rights* 18, no. 1 (2016): 167–179.

4. P. Piot, J.-J. Muyembe, and W. J. Edmunds, "Ebola in West Africa: From Disease Outbreak to Humanitarian Crisis," *Lancet Infectious Diseases* 14, no. 11 (2014): 1034–1035.

5. S. Baize, D. Pannetier, L. Oestereich, et al., "Emergence of Zaire Ebola Virus Disease in Guinea," *New England Journal of Medicine* 371, no. 15 (2014): 1418–1425; M. Hussain, "Hunger and Frustration Grow at Ebola Ground Zero in Guinea," Reuters, 2015.

6. S. Moon, D. Sridhar, M. A. Pate, et al., "Will Ebola Change the Game? Ten Essential Reforms before the Next Pandemic; The Report of the Harvard-LSHTM Independent Panel on the Global Response to Ebola," *Lancet* 386, no. 10009 (2015): 2204–2221.

7. M. Foucault, *Discipline and Punish: The Birth of the Prison* (New York: Knopf Doubleday, 1979); G. Gutiérrez, *Ciencia—cultura y dependencia* (Buenos Aires: Editorial Guadalupe, 1974).

8. D. Chandler, *Semiotics: The Basics* (Oxford: Routledge, 2002).

9. R. Braidotti, *The Posthuman* (Cambridge: Polity, 2013).

10. G. Ritzer and B. Smart, eds., *Handbook of Social Theory* (London: SAGE, 2001).

11. A. Kamradt-Scott, "WHO's to Blame? The World Health Organization and the 2014 Ebola Outbreak in West Africa," *Third World Quarterly* 37, no. 3 (2016): 401–418.

12. Médecins Sans Frontières, "Pushed to the Limit and Beyond: A Year into the Largest Ever Ebola Outbreak," March 23, 2015, https://www.msf.org/ebola-pushed-limit-and-beyond; S. Walsh, O. Johnson, *Getting to Zero: A Doctor and a Diplomat on the Ebola Frontline* (London: Zed Books, 2018).

13. J. T. Crane, *Scrambling for Africa: AIDS, Expertise, and the Rise of American Global Health Science* (Ithaca: Cornell University Press, 2013).

14. World Health Organization, "Who We Are, What We Do; About WHO," 2018 (cited January 28, 2018), http://www.who.int/about/en/.

15. P. E. Farmer, J. Bayona, M. Becerra, et al., "The Dilemma of MDR-TB in the Global Era," *International Journal of Tuberculosis and Lung Disease* 2, no. 11 (1998): 869–876.

16. P. E. Farmer, "Social Medicine and the Challenge of Biosocial Research," in Farmer, *Partner to the Poor*, 248–266.

17. Scientific Panel of the Working Group on DOTS-Plus for MDR-TB, World Health Organization, Geneva, 2000.

18. WHO Ebola Response Team, "After Ebola in West Africa—Unpredictable Risks, Preventable Epidemics," *New England Journal of Medicine* 375, no. 6 (2016): 587–596.

19. M. E. J. Woolhouse, C. Dye, J.-F. Etard, et al., "Heterogeneities in the Transmission of Infectious Agents: Implications for the Design of Control Programs," *Proceedings of the National Academy of Sciences* 94, no. 1 (1997): 338–342.

20. H. L. Dreyfus and P. Rabinow, *Michel Foucault: Beyond Structuralism and Hermeneutics*, 2nd ed. (Chicago: University of Chicago Press, 1983).

21. E. T. Richardson, M. B. Barrie, C. T. Nutt, et al., "The Ebola Suspect's Dilemma," *Lancet Global Health* 5, no. 3 (2017): e254–e256; D. Graeber, *Fragments of an Anarchist Anthropology* (Chicago: Prickly Paradigm Press, 2004).

22. H. Marcuse, *One-Dimensional Man: Studies in the Ideology of Advanced Industrial Society*, 2nd ed. (Boston: Beacon Press, 1991).

23. R. Frankfurter, M. Kardas-Nelson, A. Benton, et al., "Indirect Rule Redux: The Political Economy of Diamond Mining and Its Relation to the Ebola Outbreak in Kono District, Sierra Leone," *Review of African Political Economy* 45, no. 158 (2018): 522–540.

24. R. Levins and R. Lewontin, *The Dialectical Biologist* (Cambridge, MA: Harvard University Press, 1985).

25. P. E. Farmer, *Fevers, Feuds, and Diamonds: Ebola and the Ravages of History* (New York: Farrar, Straus and Giroux, 2020); J. Greene, M. T. Basilico, H. Kim, and P. Farmer, "Colonial Medicine and Its Legacies," in *Reimagining Global Health: An Introduction*, ed. P. Farmer, A. Kleinman, J. Y. Kim, and M. Basilico (Berkeley: University of California Press, 2013).

26. A. Leligdowicz, M. A. Fischer, T. M. Uyeki, et al., "Ebola Virus Disease and Critical Illness," *Critical Care* 20, no. 1 (2016): 217.

27. D. Fassin, *Humanitarian Reason: A Moral History of the Present* (Berkeley: University of California Press, 2011); F. Lamontagne, R. A. Fowler, N. K. Adhikari, et al., "Evidence-Based Guidelines for Supportive Care

of Patients with Ebola Virus Disease," *Lancet* 391, no. 10121 (2018): P700–P708.

28. UN Mission for Ebola Emergency Response (UNMEER), "External Situation Reports," 2014 (cited January 28, 2018), http://ebolaresponse .un.org/situation-reports?page=5; WHO Ebola Response Team, "West African Ebola Epidemic after One Year—Slowing but Not Yet under Control," *New England Journal of Medicine* 372, no. 6 (2015): 584–587.

29. C. Losson, "Ebola: A Challenge to Our Humanitarian Identity; A Letter to the MSF Movement," *Libération*, 2015 (cited April 1, 2017), http://www.liberation.fr/terre/2015/02/03/parfois-le-traitement -symptomatique-a-ete-neglige-voire-oublie_1194960.

30. Quoted from M. Lock and V.-K. Nguyen, *An Anthropology of Biomedicine* (Chichester: Wiley-Blackwell, 2010).

31. World Health Organization, "Epidemiology" (2018), http://www9 .who.int/topics/epidemiology/en/.

32. D. Freedman, *Statistical Models and Causal Inference: A Dialogue with the Social Sciences* (Cambridge: Cambridge University Press, 2010).

33. J. Ferguson, *Global Shadows: Africa in the Neoliberal World Order* (Durham: Duke University Press, 2006); D. N. McCloskey, *The Rhetoric of Economics* (Madison: University of Wisconsin Press, 1998); R. Wallace, review of Paul Richards, *Ebola: How a People's Science Helped End an Epidemic*, 2018 (cited January 25, 2018), https://antipodefoundation.org/ 2018/01/25/wallace-book-review-ebola/.

34. W. S. Y. Lau, B. D. Dalziel, S. Funk, et al., "Spatial and Temporal Dynamics of Superspreading Events in the 2014–2015 West Africa Ebola Epidemic," *Proceedings of the National Academy of Sciences* 114, no. 9 (2017): 2337–2342.

35. Foucault, *Discipline and Punish*.

36. D. J. Haraway, "A Cyborg Manifesto: Science, Technology, and Socialist Feminism in the Late Twentieth Century," in *Simians, Cyborgs, and Women: The Reinvention of Nature* (London: Free Association Books, 1991), 149–181.

37. J. Derrida, *Writing and Difference* (New York: Routledge, 2001).

38. Keshavjee, *Blind Spot.*

39. W. Rodney, *How Europe Underdeveloped Africa* (London: Bogle-L'Ouverture, 1972); S. Amin, *Neo-colonialism in West Africa* (New York: Monthly Review Press, 1973); Richardson et al., "The Ebola Suspect's Dilemma"; A. Césaire, *Discourse on Colonialism* (New York: Monthly Review Press, 1972); E. Akyeampong, R. H. Bates, N. Nunn, and J. A. Robinson, eds., *Africa's Development in Historical Perspective* (Cambridge: Cambridge University Press, 2014); J. Y. Kim, J. V. Millen, A. Irwin, and J. Gershman, eds., *Dying for Growth: Global Inequality and the Health of the Poor* (Monroe, ME: Common Courage Press, 2002); Jubilee Debt Campaign, "Honest Accounts: How the World Profits from Africa's Wealth" (London, 2017); A. Benton, "What's the Matter Boss, We Sick? A Meditation on Ebola's Origin Stories," in *Ebola's Message: Public Health and Medicine in the Twenty-First Century*, ed. N. G. Evans, T. C. Smith, and M. S. Majumder (Cambridge, MA: MIT Press, 2017); M. Karenga, "The Ethics of Reparations: Engaging the Holocaust of Enslavement," paper delivered at the National Coalition of Blacks for Reparations in America (N'COBRA) Convention (Baton Rouge, 2001), available at http://www.ncobraonline.org/wp-content/uploads/2016/02/karenga-the-ethics-of-reparations.pdf.

40. S. Abimbola, "The Foreign Gaze: Authorship in Academic Global Health," *BMJ Global Health* 4, no. 5 (2019): e002068.

41. E. W. Said, *Culture and Imperialism* (New York: Pantheon, 1993).

42. Lau et al., "Spatial and Temporal Dynamics of Superspreading Events in the 2014–2015 West Africa Ebola Epidemic."

43. World Health Organization, *Consensus Document on the Epidemiology of Severe Acute Respiratory Syndrome (SARS)* (Geneva: WHO, 2003).

44. Jubilee Debt Campaign, "Honest Accounts: How the World Profits from Africa's Wealth" (London, 2017).

45. Frankfurter et al., "Indirect Rule Redux."

46. A. Pandey, K. E. K. Atkins, I. Medlock, et al., "Strategies for Containing Ebola in West Africa," *Science* 346, no. 6212 (2014): 991–995.

47. N. Bacaër, "McKendrick and Kermack on Epidemic Modelling (1926–1927)," in *A Short History of Mathematical Population Dynamics* (London: Springer-Verlag, 2011).

48. E. T. Richardson, "Research on Oral Pre-Exposure Prophylaxis in Sub-Saharan Africa Is an Example of Biomedical Tunnel Vision," *AIDS* 28, no. 10 (2014): 1537–1538; T. S. Kuhn, *The Structure of Scientific Revolutions*, 3rd ed. (Chicago: University of Chicago Press; 1996).

49. A. Carrel, *L'homme, cet inconnu* (Paris: Plon, 1935).

50. P. E. Farmer and L. C. Ivers, "Cholera in Haiti: The Equity Agenda and the Future of Tropical Medicine," *American Journal of Tropical Medicine and Hygiene* 86, no. 1 (2012): 7–8.

51. R. Wallace, "Black Mirror: Did Neoliberal Epidemiology Impose Its Image Upon Ebola's Epicenter?," *Antipode*, 2018 (cited January 29, 2018), https://radicalantipode.files.wordpress.com/2018/01/book-review _wallace-on-richards1.pdf.

52. J. Biehl, "Theorizing Global Health," *Medicine Anthropology Theory* 3, no. 2 (2016): 127–142.

53. For a discussion of path-dependent government corruption and its relation to colonial indirect-rule strategies, see D. Acemoglu, I. N. Chaves, P. Osafo-Kwaako, and J. A. Robinson, "Indirect Rule and State Weakness in Africa: Sierra Leone in Comparative Perspective," in *African Successes*, vol. 4: *Sustainable Growth*, ed. S. Edwards, S. Johnson, and D. Weil (Chicago: University of Chicago Press, 2016), 343–370.

54. E. T. Richardson, J. D. Kelly, O. Sesay, et al., "The Symbolic Violence of 'Outbreak': A Mixed-Methods, Quasi-Experimental Impact Evaluation of Social Protection on Ebola Survivor Wellbeing," *Social Science and Medicine* 195 (2017): 77–82; M. Ani, *Let the Circle Be Unbroken: The Implications of African Spirituality in the Diaspora* (Trenton, NJ: Red Sea Press, 1994); M. Karenga, *Introduction to Black Studies* (Los Angeles: University of Sankore Press, 1993).

55. C. L. Briggs, "Why Nation-States and Journalists Can't Teach People to Be Healthy: Power and Pragmatic Miscalculation in Public Discourses on Health," *Medical Anthropology Quarterly* 17 (2003): 287–321.

Redescription 5

1. D. Swartz, *Culture and Power: The Sociology of Pierre Bourdieu* (Chicago: University of Chicago Press, 1997).

2. E. T. Richardson, M. B. Barrie, C. T. Nutt, et al., "The Ebola Suspect's Dilemma," *Lancet Global Health* 5, no. 3 (2017): e254–e256.

3. Richardson et al., "The Ebola Suspect's Dilemma"; E. T. Richardson, M. P. Fallah, J. D. Kelly, and M. B. Barrie, "The Predicament of Patients with Suspected Ebola—Authors' Reply," *Lancet Global Health* 5, no. 7 (2017): e660–e661; R. Colebunders, S. T. Jacob, and J. van Griensven, "The Predicament of Patients with Suspected Ebola," *Lancet Global Health* 5, no. 7 (2017): e658; T. Mayrhofer, R. M. Hamm, J. Van den Ende, I. Hozo, and B. Djulbegovic, "The Predicament of Patients with Suspected Ebola," *Lancet Global Health* 5, no. 7 (2017): e657; F. Fitzgerald, D. E. Baion, K. Wing, S. Yeung, and F. Sahr, "The Predicament of Patients with Suspected Ebola," *Lancet Global Health* 5, no. 7 (2017): e659.

4. A. Rubinstein, *Economic Fables* (Cambridge: Open Book, 2012).

5. P. Bourdieu, *Language and Symbolic Power* (Cambridge, MA: Harvard University Press, 1991).

Redescription 6

1. W. D. Mignolo and C. W. Walsh, *On Decoloniality: Concepts, Analytics, Praxis* (Durham: Duke University Press, 2018).

2. C. Anderson, "The End of Theory: The Data Deluge Makes the Scientific Method Obsolete," *Wired*, June 23, 2008.

3. S. Zuboff, *The Age of Surveillance Capitalism: The Fight for a Human Future at the New Frontier of Power* (New York: PublicAffairs, 2019); D.

Lazer, A. Pentland, L. Adamic, et al., "Computational Social Science," *Science* 323, no. 5915 (2009): 721–723.

4. S. Bansal, G. Chowell, L. Simonsen, A. Vespignani, and C. Viboud, "Big Data for Infectious Disease Surveillance and Modeling," *Journal of Infectious Diseases* 214, suppl. 4 (2016): 375–379.

5. L. H. Malkki, *The Need to Help: The Domestic Arts of International Humanitarianism* (Durham: Duke University Press, 2015).

6. F. Manji and C. O'Coill, "The Missionary Position: NGOs and Development in Africa," *International Affairs* 78, no. 3 (2002): 567–583.

7. N. C. Grassly and C. Fraser, "Mathematical Models of Infectious Disease Transmission," *Nature Reviews Microbiology* 6 (2008): 477.

8. A. T. Fojo, E. A. Kendall, P. Kasaie, S. Shrestha, T. A. Louis, and D. W. Dowdy, "Mathematical Modeling of 'Chronic' Infectious Diseases: Unpacking the Black Box," *Open Forum Infectious Diseases* 4, no. 4 (2017): ofx172.

9. J.-P. Chretien, S. Riley, and D. B. George, "Mathematical Modeling of the West Africa Ebola Epidemic," *eLife* 4 (2015): e09186.

10. M. Meltzer, C. Atkins, S. Santibanez, et al., "Estimating the Future Number of Cases in the Ebola Epidemic—Liberia and Sierra Leone, 2014–2015," *Morbidity and Mortality Weekly Report* 63, no. 3 (2015).

11. M. Stobbe, "CDC's Top Modeler Courts Controversy with Disease Estimate," Associated Press, 2015; S. M. McDonald, *Ebola: A Big Data Disaster* (Delhi: Centre for Internet and Society, 2016).

12. G. E. P. Box, "Robustness in the Strategy of Scientific Model Building," Technical Summary Report #1954, Mathematics Research Center, University of Wisconsin-Madison, 1979.

13. J. P. A. Ioannidis, "Why Most Clinical Research Is Not Useful," *PLOS Medicine* 13, no. 6 (2016): e1002049.

14. A. H. Kelly and L. McGoey, "Facts, Power and Global Evidence: A New Empire of Truth," *Economy and Society* 47, no. 1 (2018): 1–26.

15. J. Go, *Postcolonial Thought and Social Theory* (New York: Oxford University Press, 2016); M. Trouillot, *Silencing the Past: Power and the Production of History* (Boston: Beacon Press, 1995).

16. P. E. Farmer, *Pathologies of Power: Health, Human Rights, and the New War on the Poor*, 2nd ed. (Berkeley: University of California Press, 2005); J. Galtung, "Kulturelle Gewalt," *Der Bürger im Staat* 43 (1993): 106; P. E. Farmer, *Infections and Inequalities: The Modern Plagues* (Berkeley: University of California Press, 2001); P. E. Farmer, B. Nizeye, S. Stulac, and S. Keshavjee, "Structural Violence and Clinical Medicine," *PLoS Medicine* 3, no. 10 (2006): 1686–1691; N. Scheper-Hughes, *Death without Weeping: Violence of Everyday Life in Brazil* (Berkeley: University of California Press, 1993).

17. E. T. Richardson, M. B. Barrie, J. D. Kelly, Y. Dibba, S. Koedoyoma, and P. E. Farmer, "Biosocial Approaches to the 2013–16 Ebola Pandemic," *Health and Human Rights* 18, no. 1 (2016): 167–179; P. E. Farmer, "Social Inequalities and Emerging Infectious Diseases," *Emerging Infectious Diseases* 2, no. 4 (1996): 259–269; I. Abdullah and I. Rashid, eds., *Understanding West Africa's Ebola Epidemic: Towards a Political Economy* (London: Zed Books, 2017); E. T. Richardson, J. D. Kelly, O. Sesay, et al., "The Symbolic Violence of 'Outbreak': A Mixed-Methods, Quasi-Experimental Impact Evaluation of Social Protection on Ebola Survivor Wellbeing," *Social Science and Medicine* 195 (2017): 77–82; M. Leach, "Haemorrhagic Fevers in Africa: Narratives, Politics and Pathways of Disease and Response," *Wellcome History* 38 (2008): 7–9; A. Wilkinson and M. Leach, "Briefing: Ebola—Myths, Realities, and Structural Violence," *African Affairs* 114 (August 2014): 136–148; R. G. Wallace, M. Gilbert, R. Wallace, C. Pittiglio, R. Mattioli, and R. Kock, "Did Ebola Emerge in West Africa by a Policy-Driven Phase Change in Agroecology?," *Environment and Planning A* 46 (2014): 2533–2542; S. A. Abramowitz, K. E. McLean, S. L. McKune, et al., "Community-Centered Responses to Ebola in Urban Liberia: The View from Below," *PLOS Neglected Tropical Diseases* 9, no. 4 (2015): e0003706; A. Benton and K. Y. Dionne, "International Political Economy and the 2014 West African Ebola Outbreak," *African Studies Review* 58, no. 1 (2015): 223–236; J. D. Kelly, E. T. Richardson, M. Drasher, et al., "Food Insecurity as a Risk Factor for Outcomes Related

to Ebola Virus Disease in Kono District, Sierra Leone: A Cross-Sectional Study," *American Journal of Tropical Medicine and Hygiene* 98, no. 5 (2018): 1484–1488.

18. T. S. Kuhn, *The Structure of Scientific Revolutions*, 3rd ed. (Chicago: University of Chicago Press, 1996).

19. J. S. Nelson, A. Megill, and D. N. McCloskey, "Rhetoric of Inquiry," in *The Rhetoric of the Human Sciences: Language and Argument in Scholarship and Public Affairs*, ed. J. S. Nelson, A. Megill, and D. N. McCloskey (Madison: University of Wisconsin Press, 1987), 3–18; P. Feyerabend, *Against Method*, 4th ed. (New York: Verso, 2010).

20. A. Giddens, *New Rules of Sociological Method*, 2nd ed. (Cambridge: Polity, 1993).

21. McDonald, *Ebola: A Big Data Disaster*.

22. M. Taussig, *The Devil and Commodity Fetishism in South America*, 2nd ed. (Chapel Hill: University of North Carolina Press, 2010); M. Vaughan, *Curing Their Ills: Colonial Power and African Illness* (Redwood City: Stanford University Press, 1991).

23. Farmer, *Pathologies of Power*; E. T. Richardson, M. B. Barrie, C. T. Nutt, et al., "The Ebola Suspect's Dilemma," *Lancet Global Health* 5, no. 3 (2017); E. T. Richardson, M. P. Fallah, J. D. Kelly, and M. B. Barrie, "The Predicament of Patients with Suspected Ebola—Authors' Reply," *Lancet Global Health* 5, no. 7 (2017); D. Fassin, *When Bodies Remember: Experiences and Politics of AIDS in South Africa* (Berkeley: University of California Press, 2007).

24. J. Hickel, *The Divide: Global Inequality from Conquest to Free Markets* (New York: W. W. Norton, 2018); J. Ferguson, *Global Shadows: Africa in the Neoliberal World Order* (Durham: Duke University Press, 2006); J. Ferguson and L. Lohmann, "The Anti-Politics Machine: 'Development' and Bureaucratic Power in Lesotho," *Ecologist* 24, no. 5 (1994): 176–181.

25. M. Leach and I. Scoones, "The Social and Political Lives of Zoonotic Disease Models: Narratives, Science and Policy," *Social Science and Medicine* 88 (2013): 10–17.

26. R. Virchow, "Der Armenarzt," *Medicinische Reform* 18 (1848): 125–127.

27. L. M. Morgan, "Dependency Theory in the Political Economy of Health: An Anthropological Critique," *Medical Anthropology Quarterly* 1, no. 2 (1987): 131–154; L. Doyal, *The Political Economy of Health* (Boston: South End Press, 1979).

28. F. Fanon, *Black Skin, White Masks* (Boston: Grove Press, 1967).

29. G. S. Coulthard, "Subjects of Empire: Indigenous Peoples and the 'Politics of Recognition' in Canada," *Contemporary Political Theory* 6 (2007): 437–460.

30. F. Fanon, *The Wretched of the Earth* (New York: Grove Press, 2005).

31. L.-Q. Fang, Y. Yang, J.-F. Jiang, et al., "Transmission Dynamics of Ebola Virus Disease and Intervention Effectiveness in Sierra Leone," *Proceedings of the National Academy of Sciences* 113, no. 16 (2016): 4488–4493.

32. L. T. Smith, *Decolonizing Methodologies: Research and Indigenous Peoples* (London: Zed Books, 2012).

33. Coulthard, "Subjects of Empire"; G. B. Tangwa, A. Abayomi, S. J. Ujewe, and N. S. Munung, eds., *Socio-cultural Dimensions of Emerging Infectious Diseases in Africa: An Indigenous Response to Deadly Epidemics* (Cham: Springer, 2019); S. Abimbola, "The Foreign Gaze: Authorship in Academic Global Health," *BMJ Global Health* 4, no. 5 (2019): e002068.

34. J. B. Aristide, *Aristide and the Endless Revolution* (film, 2005).

35. P. E. Farmer, "Douze points en faveur de la restitution à Haïti de la dette française," 2003, http://www.ijdh.org/2010/03/topics/economy/restitution-of-haitis-independence-debt/; H. M. Beckles, *Britain's Black Debt: Reparations for Caribbean Slavery and Native Genocide* (Kingston: University of the West Indies Press, 2013); W. A. Darity and A. K. Mullen, *From Here to Equality: Reparations for Black Americans in the Twenty-First Century* (Chapel Hill: University of North Carolina Press, 2020); T.-N. Coates, "The Case for Reparations," *Atlantic* (June 2014); K.

Franke, *Repair: Redeeming the Promise of Abolition* (Chicago: Haymarket Books, 2019).

36. C. M. Peak, A. Wesolowski, E. zu Erbach-Schoenberg, et al., "Population Mobility Reductions Associated with Travel Restrictions during the Ebola Epidemic in Sierra Leone: Use of Mobile Phone Data," *International Journal of Epidemiology* 47 (2018): 1–9.

37. S. L. Erikson, *Cell Phones as an Anticipatory Technology: Behind the Hype of Big Data for Ebola Detection* (Halle: German Research Foundation, 2018)

38. V. Adams, "Subjects, Profits, Erasures," in *When People Come First: Critical Studies in Global Health*, ed. J. Biehl and A. Petryna (Princeton: Princeton University Press, 2013), 79.

39. A. Maxmen, "Surveillance Science," *Nature* 569 (2019): 614–617.

40. Benton and Dionne, "International Political Economy and the 2014 West African Ebola Outbreak."

41. Jubilee Debt Campaign, "Honest Accounts: How the World Profits from Africa's Wealth" (London, 2017).

42. J. Biehl and A. Petryna, "Critical Global Health," in Biehl and Petryna, *When People Come First.*

43. M. Weber, *The Protestant Ethic and the Spirit of Capitalism*, 2nd ed. (London: Routledge, 2001).

44. B. Agger, *Critical Social Theories* (Boulder: Paradigm, 2006).

45. V. Adams, ed., *Metrics: What Counts in Global Health* (Durham: Duke University Press, 2016).

46. A. Kleinman, V. Das, and M. Lock, eds., *Social Suffering* (Berkeley: University of California Press, 1997); P. Bourgois and J. Schonberg, *Righteous Dopefiend* (Berkeley: University of California Press, 2009).

47. Fojo et al., "Mathematical Modeling of 'Chronic' Infectious Diseases."

48. Radical Statistics Group, "About" (cited August 22, 2018), http://www.radstats.org.uk/about-radical-statistics/; L. A. Avilés, "Epidemiology as Discourse: The Politics of Development Institutions in the Epidemiological Profile of El Salvador," *Journal of Epidemiology and Community Health* 55 (2001): 164–171; J. Breilh, *Epidemiología Crítica: Ciencia Emancipadora e Interculturalidad* (Buenos Aires: Lugar Editorial, 2003).

49. J. Breilh, "Latin American Critical ('Social') Epidemiology: New Settings for an Old Dream," *International Journal of Epidemiology* 37 (2008): 745–750.

50. A. Cerón, "Neocolonial Epidemiology: Public Health Practice and the Right to Health in Guatemala," *Medicine Anthropology Theory* 6, no. 1 (2019): 30–54.

51. M. P. Fallah, L. A. Skrip, S. Gertler, D. Yamin, and A. P. Galvani, "Quantifying Poverty as a Driver of Ebola Transmission," *PLOS Neglected Tropical Diseases* 9, no. 12 (2016): e0004260.

52. P. E. Farmer, "An Anthropology of Structural Violence," *Current Anthropology* 45, no. 3 (2004): 305–325.

53. M. Foucault, *Discipline and Punish: The Birth of the Prison* (New York: Knopf Doubleday, 1979).

54. J. T. Crane, *Scrambling for Africa: AIDS, Expertise, and the Rise of American Global Health Science* (Ithaca: Cornell University Press, 2013); P. J. Hountondji, "Recapturing," in *The Surreptitious Speech: Présence Africaine and the Politics of Otherness, 1947–1987*, ed. V. Y. Mudimbe (Chicago: University of Chicago Press; 1992), 238–248.

55. Vandana Shiva, *The Monocultures of the Mind: Perspectives in Biodiversity* (London: Zed Books; 1993).

56. M. Karenga, "The Ethics of Reparations: Engaging the Holocaust of Enslavement," paper delivered at the National Coalition of Blacks for Reparations in America (N'COBRA) convention (Baton Rouge, 2001), available at http://www.ncobraonline.org/wp-content/uploads/2016/02/karenga-the-ethics-of-reparations.pdf; Richardson et al., "The Symbolic Violence of 'Outbreak'"; M. Ani, *Let the Circle Be Unbroken: The*

Implications of African Spirituality in the Diaspora (Trenton, NJ: Red Sea Press, 1994).

57. A. Césaire, *Discourse on Colonialism* (New York: Monthly Review Press, 1972).

58. W. Rodney, *How Europe Underdeveloped Africa* (London: Bogle-L'Ouverture, 1972); S. Amin, *Neo-colonialism in West Africa* (New York: Monthly Review Press, 1973); E. Akyeampong, R. H. Bates, N. Nunn, and J. A. Robinson, eds., *Africa's Development in Historical Perspective* (Cambridge: Cambridge University Press, 2014); A. G. Frank, "The Development of Underdevelopment," *Monthly Review* 18, no. 4 (1966): 17–31; M. Turshen, "The Impact of Colonialism on Health and Health Services in Tanzania," *International Journal of Health Services* 7, no. 1 (1977): 7–35.

59. J. Y. Kim, J. V. Millen, A. Irwin, and J. Gershman, eds., *Dying for Growth: Global Inequality and the Health of the Poor* (Monroe, ME: Common Courage Press, 2002).

60. H. Brown and A. H. Kelly, "Material Proximities and Hotspots: Toward an Anthropology of Viral Hemorrhagic Fevers," *Medical Anthropology Quarterly* 28, no. 2 (2014): 280–303; A. B. Zack-Williams, "Diamond Mining and Underdevelopment in Sierra Leone, 1930/1980," *Africa Development* 15, no 2 (1990): 95–117; G. Mitman and P. Erickson, "Latex and Blood," *Radical History Review* 107 (2010): 45–73.

61. Jubilee Debt Campaign, "Honest Accounts"; J. Hickel, "The Development Delusion: Foreign Aid and Inequality," *American Affairs* 1, no. 3 (2017); Z. Cope, *The Wealth of (Some) Nations: Imperialism and the Mechanics of Value Transfer* (London: Pluto Press; 2019).

62. N. Fraser, *Unruly Practices: Power, Discourse, and Gender in Contemporary Social Theory* (Minneapolis: University of Minnesota Press, 1989); E. T. Richardson, S. E. Collins, T. Kung, et al., "Gender Inequality and HIV Transmission: A Global Analysis," *Journal of the International AIDS Society* 17 (2014): 19035; G. S. Gonsalves, E. H. Kaplan, and A. D. Paltiel, "Reducing Sexual Violence by Increasing the Supply of Toilets in Khayelitsha, South Africa: A Mathematical Model," *PLOS ONE* 10, no. 4 (2015): e0122244, https://doi.org/10.1371/journal.pone.0122244.

63. Frankfurter et al., "Indirect Rule Redux."

64. A. R. Thomas, "President Bio Wants Diamonds to Be Cut and Polished in Sierra Leone," *Sierra Leone Telegraph* (2018), https://www.thesierraleonetelegraph.com/president-bio-wants-diamonds-to-be-cut-and-polished-in-sierra-leone/.

65. Sierra Leone Ministry of Health and Sanitation, *Maternal Death Surveillance and Response Annual Report* (2016); E. G. Karmbor-Ballah, M. P. Fallah, J. B. Silverstein, H. N. Gilbert, I. K. Desai, J. S. Mukherjee, P. E. Farmer, and E. T. Richardson, "Maternal Mortality and the Metempsychosis of User Fees in Liberia: A Mixed-Methods Analysis," *Scientific African* 3 (2019): e00050, doi: 10.1016/j.sciaf.2019.e00050.

66. Rodney, *How Europe Underdeveloped Africa*.

67. M. Joffe, M. Gambhir, M. Chadeau-Hyam, and P. Vineis, "Causal Diagrams in Systems Epidemiology," *Emerging Themes in Epidemiology* 9 (2012): 1.

68. A. Kleinman, *The Illness Narratives: Suffering, Healing and the Human Condition* (New York: Basic Books, 1988).

69. J. Pearl and D. Mackenzie, *The Book of Why: The New Science of Cause and Effect* (New York: Basic Books, 2018), 113.

70. M. A. Hernán, S. Hernández-Díaz, M. M. Werler, and A. A. Mitchell, "Causal Knowledge as a Prerequisite for Confounding Evaluation: An Application to Birth Defects Epidemiology," *American Journal of Epidemiology* 155, no. 2 (2002): 176–184.

71. P. Robbins, *Political Ecology: A Critical Introduction*, 2nd ed. (West Sussex: John Wiley, 2012); J. Mayer, "Geography, Ecology and Emerging Infectious Diseases," *Social Science and Medicine* 50, no. 7–8 (2000): 937–952.

72. W. Easterly, *The Tyranny of Experts: Economists, Dictators, and the Forgotten Rights of the Poor* (New York: Basic Books, 2013); A. Escobar, *Encountering Development: The Making and Unmaking of the Third World* (Princeton: Princeton University Press, 2011).

73. S. Schwartz, S. J. Prins, U. B. Campbell, and N. M. Gatto, "Is the 'Well-Defined Intervention Assumption' Politically Conservative?," *Social Science and Medicine* 166 (2016): 254–257.

74. L. Althusser, "Ideology and Ideological State Apparatuses," in *Lenin and Philosophy and other Essays* (New York: Monthly Review Press, 1971); M. Horkheimer and T. W. Adorno, *Dialectic of Enlightenment* (New York: Herder and Herder; 1972); D. Leopold, "Marxism and Ideology: From Marx to Althusser," in *The Oxford Handbook of Political Ideologies*, ed. M. Freeden and M. Stears (Oxford: Oxford University Press, 2013); P. A. Braveman, "Epidemiology and (Neo-) Colonialism," *Journal of Epidemiology and Community Health* 55 (2001): 160–161; S. Hall, *Cultural Studies 1983: A Theoretical History* (Durham: Duke University Press, 2016).

75. B. N. Patenaude, N. Chimbindi, D. Pillay, and T. Bärnighausen, "The Impact of ART Initiation on Household Food Security over Time," *Social Science and Medicine* 198 (2018): 175–184.

76. Schwartz et al., "Is the 'Well-Defined Intervention Assumption' Politically Conservative?"

77. C. J. Ruhm, "Shackling the Identification Police," National Bureau of Economics Research Working Paper 25320 (2018).

78. Ruhm, *Shackling the Identification Police*.

79. See T. Pogge, *World Poverty and Human Rights*, 2nd ed. (Cambridge: Polity, 2008), for a description of the sophisticated means by which individuals exploit moral loopholes and other methods of morality avoidance. For a discussion of objectivity vs. solidarity and the correlative attempt to avoid facing up to contingency, see Pogge, *World Poverty and Human Rights*, and R. Rorty, "Solidarity or Objectivity?," in *Relativism: Interpretation and Confrontation*, ed. M. Krausz (Notre Dame: University of Notre Dame Press, 1989), 167–183.

80. J. Aldred, *Licence to Be Bad: How Economics Corrupted Us* (London: Allen Lane, 2019).

81. I. M. Young, *Responsibility for Justice* (Oxford: Oxford University Press, 2011).

82. A. Giridharadas, *Winners Take All: The Elite Charade of Changing the World* (New York: Knopf, 2018); S. Žižek, *Violence: Six Sideways Reflections* (New York: Picador, 2008); L. McGoey, *No Such Thing as a Free Gift* (London: Verso, 2015).

83. T. Burgis, *The Looting Machine: Warlords, Oligarchs, Corporations, Smugglers, and the Theft of Africa's Wealth* (New York: Public Affairs, 2016).

84. Hickel, *The Divide*.

85. D. Butler, "World's Foremost Institute on Death and Disease Metrics Gets Massive Cash Boost," *Nature* (2017), https://www.nature.com/news/world-s-foremost-institute-on-death-and-disease-metrics-gets-massive-cash-boost-1.21373.

86. J. S. Kaufman and R. S. Cooper, "Seeking Causal Explanations in Social Epidemiology," *American Journal of Epidemiology* 150, no. 2 (1999): 113–120.

87. S. S. Lim, T. Vos, A. D. Flaxman, et al., "A Comparative Risk Assessment of Burden of Disease and Injury Attributable to 67 Risk Factors and Risk Factor Clusters in 21 Regions, 1990–2010: A Systematic Analysis for the Global Burden of Disease Study 2010," *Lancet* 380, no. 9859 (2012): 2224–2260.

88. G. Pohlhaus Jr., "Relational Knowing and Epistemic Injustice: Toward a Theory of Willful Hermeneutical Ignorance," *Hypatia* 27, no. 4 (2012): 715–735.

89. L. Boltanski, *On Critique: A Sociology of Emancipation* (Cambridge: Polity, 2011).

90. T. J. Csordas, "Embodiment as a Paradigm for Anthropology," *Ethos* 18, no. 1 (1990): 5–47; N. Krieger, "Theories for Social Epidemiology in the 21st Century: An Ecosocial Perspective," *International Journal of Epidemiology* 30, no. 4 (2001): 668–677.

91. S. Keshavjee, *Blind Spot: How Neoliberalism Infiltrated Global Health* (Berkeley: University of California Press, 2014).

92. H.-K. Trask, *From a Native Daughter: Colonialism and Sovereignty in Hawai'i* (Honolulu: University of Hawai'i Press, 1999).

93. M. Rigby, S. Deshpande, and M. Blair, "Another Blow to Credibility in Published Data Sources," *Lancet* 394, no. 10192 (2019): 26–27.

94. S. Anand and K. Hanson, "Disability Adjusted Life Years: A Critical Perspective," *Journal of Health Economics* 16, no. 6 (1997): 685–702; A. Becker, A. Motgi, J. Weigel, G. Raviola, S. Keshavjee, and A. Kleinman, "The Unique Challenges of Mental Health and MDRTB: Critical Perspectives on Metrics of Disease Burden," in *Reimagining Global Health: An Introduction*, ed. P. Farmer, A. Kleinman, J. Y. Kim, and M. Basilico (Berkeley: University of California Press, 2013).

95. A. Kleinman, *Writing at the Margin: Discourse between Anthropology and Medicine* (Berkeley: University of California Press, 1995).

96. A. J. McMichael, "Prisoners of the Proximate: Loosening the Constraints on Epidemiology in an Age of Change," *American Journal of Epidemiology* 149, no. 10 (1999): 887–897.

97. Breilh, *Epidemiología Crítica*; M. C. Inhorn and P. J. Brown, *The Anthropology of Infectious Disease: International Health Perspectives* (London: Routledge, 1997).

98. J. Mayer, "The Political Ecology of Disease as One New Focus for Medical Geography," *Progress in Human Geography* 20, no. 4 (1996): 441–456.

99. M. Susser and E. Susser, "Choosing a Future for Epidemiology: I. Eras and Paradigms," *American Journal of Public Health* 86, no. 5 (1996): 668–673.

100. J. Medina, *The Epistemology of Resistance: Gender and Racial Oppression, Epistemic Injustice, and the Social Imagination* (Oxford: Oxford University Press, 2013); N. Scheper-Hughes, "Three Propositions for a Critically Applied Medical Anthropology," *Social Science and Medicine* 30, no. 2 (1990): 189–197.

101. P. Vannini, "Critical Pragmatism," in L. M. Given, ed., *The Sage Encyclopedia of Qualitative Research Methods* (Thousand Oaks, CA: SAGE Publications, 2008): 160–164.

102. V. Dalmiya, *Caring to Know: Comparative Care Ethics, Feminist Epistemology, and the Mahābhārata* (Oxford: Oxford University Press, 2016).

Redescription 7

1. D. Swartz, *Culture and Power: The Sociology of Pierre Bourdieu* (Chicago: University of Chicago Press, 1997); M. Emirbayer, "Manifesto for a Relational Sociology," *American Journal of Sociology* 103, no. 2 (1997): 281–317; P. Bourdieu and L. I. D. Wacquant, *An Invitation to Reflexive Sociology* (Chicago: University of Chicago Press, 1992); T. L. Goldberg and J. A. Patz, "The Need for a Global Health Ethic," *Lancet* 386, no. 10007 (2015): e37–e39.

2. P. E. Farmer, "An Anthropology of Structural Violence," *Current Anthropology* 45, no. 3 (2004): 305–325.

3. A. Kleinman, *The Illness Narratives: Suffering, Healing and the Human Condition* (New York: Basic Books, 1988).

4. D. Mitchell, *Cloud Atlas: A Novel* (New York: Random House, 2004).

5. P. Vinck, P. N. Pham, K. K. Bindu, J. Bedford, and E. J. Nilles, "Institutional Trust and Misinformation in the Response to the 2018–19 Ebola Outbreak in North Kivu, DR Congo: A Population-Based Survey," *Lancet Infectious Diseases* 19, no. 5 (2019): 529–536.

6. A. Mbembe, *On the Postcolony* (Berkeley: University of California Press, 2001).

7. P. L. Berger and T. Luckmann, *The Social Construction of Reality: A Treatise in the Sociology of Knowledge* (New York: Anchor, 1967).

8. S. Fuller, "The Public Intellectual as Agent of Justice: In Search of a Regime," *Philosophy and Rhetoric* 39, no. 2 (2006): 147–156.

9. N. wa Thiong'o, *Decolonising the Mind: The Politics of Language in African Literature* (London: James Curry, 1986).

10. A. Mbembe, *Critique of Black Reason* (Durham: Duke University Press, 2017).

11. E. W. Said, *Orientalism* (New York: Vintage, 1979); M. Foucault, *Discipline and Punish: The Birth of the Prison* (New York: Knopf Doubleday, 1979); G. Gutiérrez, *Ciencia—cultura y dependencia* (Buenos Aires: Editorial Guadalupe, 1974).

12. C. W. Mills, "White Ignorance," in *Race and Epistemologies of Ignorance*, ed. S. Sullivan and N. Tuana (Albany: State University of New York Press, 2007), 11–38.

13. A. Gramsci, *Selections from the Prison Notebooks* (London: Lawrence and Wishart, 1971); S. Schwartz, S. J. Prins, U. B. Campbell, and N. M. Gatto, "Is the 'Well-Defined Intervention Assumption' Politically Conservative?," *Social Science and Medicine* 166 (2016): 254–257.

14. M. U. G. Kraemer, D. M. Pigott, S. C. Hill, et al., "Dynamics of Conflict during the Ebola Outbreak in the Democratic Republic of the Congo 2018–2019," *BMC Medicine* 18, no. 113 (2020).

15. Anonymous, "Death and Disbelievers: Ebola in West Africa," *Economist* 412, no. 8898 (2014): 36.

16. G. Pohlhaus Jr., "Relational Knowing and Epistemic Injustice: Toward a Theory of Willful Hermeneutical Ignorance," *Hypatia* 27, no. 4 (2012): 715–735.

17. E. T. Richardson, M. B. Barrie, J. D. Kelly, Y. Dibba, S. Koedoyoma, and P. E. Farmer, "Biosocial Approaches to the 2013–16 Ebola Pandemic," *Health and Human Rights* 18, no. 1 (2016): 167–179; R. Rorty, "Solidarity or Objectivity?," in *Relativism: Interpretation and Confrontation*, ed. M. Krausz (Notre Dame: University of Notre Dame Press, 1989), 167–183; P. E. Farmer, "From Haiti to Rwanda: AIDS and Accusations," in *Partner to the Poor: A Paul Farmer Reader*, ed. H. Saussy (Berkeley: University of California Press, 2010).

18. J. Habermas, *Knowledge and Human Interests*, 2nd ed. (London: Heinemann, 1978).

19. B. Agger, *Critical Social Theories* (Boulder: Paradigm, 2006).

20. J. Clammer, "Decolonizing the Mind: Schwimmer, Habermas and the Anthropology of Postcolonialism," *Anthropologica* 50, no. 1 (2008): 157–168.

21. R. Levins and R. Lewontin, *The Dialectical Biologist* (Cambridge, MA: Harvard University Press, 1985).

22. L. Polman, *The Crisis Caravan: What's Wrong with Humanitarian Aid* (London: Picador, 2010).

23. Bourdieu and Wacquant, *An Invitation to Reflexive Sociology*.

24. E. Bendavid and J. Bhattacharya, "The Relationship of Health Aid to Population Health Improvements," *JAMA Internal Medicine* 174, no. 6 (2014): 881–887.

25. Jubilee Debt Campaign, "Honest Accounts: How the World Profits from Africa's Wealth" (London, 2017).

26. A. Maxmen, "Behind the Front Lines of the Ebola Wars," *Nature*, September 11, 2019, https://www.nature.com/articles/d41586-019-02673 -7?utm_source=fbk_nnc&utm_medium=social&utm_campaign=nature news&sf219355602=1.

27. My colleagues and I have analyzed a similar dynamic in Sierra Leone. See R. Frankfurter, M. Kardas-Nelson, A. Benton, et al., "Indirect Rule Redux: The Political Economy of Diamond Mining and Its Relation to the Ebola Outbreak in Kono District, Sierra Leone," *Review of African Political Economy* 45, no. 158 (2018): 522–540.

28. A. Hochschild, "Blood and Treasure: Why One of the World's Richest Countries Is Also One of Its Poorest," *Mother Jones*, March-April 2010.

29. Vinck et al., "Institutional Trust and Misinformation in the Response to the 2018–19 Ebola Outbreak in North Kivu, DR Congo."

30. E. E. Evans-Pritchard, "The Notion of Witchcraft Explains Unfortunate Events," in *Witchcraft, Oracles and Magic among the Azande* (Oxford: Clarendon, 1976), 18–32.

31. M. C. Kasereka, J. Sawatzky, and M. T. Hawkes, "Ebola Epidemic in War-Torn Democratic Republic of Congo, 2018: Acceptability and Patient Satisfaction of the Recombinant Vesicular Stomatitis Virus–Zaire Ebolavirus Vaccine," *Vaccine* 37, no. 16 (2019): 2174–2178.

32. S. R. Lowes and E. Montero, "The Legacy of Colonial Medicine Campaigns in Central Africa," Centre for Economic Policy Research, London, 2018, CEPR Discussion Paper 12772.

33. D. R. Headrick, "Sleeping Sickness Epidemics and Colonial Responses in East and Central Africa, 1900–1940," *PLoS Neglected Tropical Diseases* 8, no. 4 (2014): e2772–e2772.

34. M. Alsan and M. Wanamaker, "Tuskegee and the Health of Black Men," *Quarterly Journal of Economics* 133, no. 1 (2017): 407–455.

35. F. Chipato, "The Political Economy of Aid in Zimbabwe," *Review of African Political Economy* (2019), http://roape.net/2019/05/09/the -political-economy-of-aid-in-zimbabwe/.

36. N. Pollack, "Failure of the American Left: Iron-Fisted Co-Optation," *CounterPunch* (2015), https://www.counterpunch.org/2015/12/18/failure -of-the-american-left-iron-fisted-co-optation/; M. Bookchin, *The Murray Bookchin Reader* (Montréal: Black Rose Books, 1999).

37. A. Mbembe, "What Is Postcolonial Thinking?," *Esprit* (December 2006).

38. R. Grosfoguel, "Decolonizing Post-Colonial Studies and Paradigms of Political-Economy: Transmodernity, Decolonial Thinking, and Global Coloniality," *Transmodernity* 1, no. 1 (2011).

Redescription 8

1. J. S. Nelson, A. Megill, and D. N. McCloskey, "Rhetoric of Inquiry," in *The Rhetoric of the Human Sciences: Language and Argument in Scholarship and Public Affairs*, ed. J. S. Nelson, A. Megill, and D. N. McCloskey (Madison: University of Wisconsin Press, 1987), 3–18; Phillip E. Agre, *Computation and Human Experience* (Cambridge: Cambridge University Press, 1997).

2. A. Maxmen, "Behind the Front Lines of the Ebola Wars," *Nature*, September 11, 2019, https://www.nature.com/articles/d41586-019-02673-7 ?utm_source=fbk_nnc&utm_medium=social&utm_campaign=naturene ws&sf219355602=1.

3. C. Latkin, M. R. Weeks, L. Glasman, C. Galletly, and D. Albarracin, "A Dynamic Social Systems Model for Considering Structural Factors in HIV Prevention and Detection," *AIDS and Behavior* 14, suppl. 2 (2010): 222–238; UNAIDS, *Combination HIV Prevention: Tailoring and Coordinating Biomedical, Behavioural and Structural Strategies to Reduce New HIV Infections* (Geneva, 2010); L. F. Berkman, I. Kawachi, and M. Glymour, eds., *Social Epidemiology* (Oxford: Oxford University Press, 2014).

4. A. Pettifor, C. Macphail, N. Nguyen, and M. Rosenberg, "Can Money Prevent the Spread of HIV? A Review of Cash Payments for HIV Prevention," *AIDS and Behavior* 16 (2012): 1729–1738.

5. B. Auvert, D. Taljaard, E. Lagarde, J. Sobngwi-Tambekou, R. Sitta, and A. Puren, "Randomized, Controlled Intervention Trial of Male Circumcision for Reduction of HIV Infection Risk: The ANRS 1265 Trial," *PLoS Medicine* 2, no. 11 (2005): e298; M. S. Cohen, Y. Q. Chen, M. McCauley, et al., "Prevention of HIV-1 Infection with Early Antiretroviral Therapy," *New England Journal of Medicine* 365, no. 6 (2011): 493–505.

6. M. C. Thigpen, P. M. Kebaabetswe, L. A. Paxton, et al., "Antiretroviral Preexposure Prophylaxis for Heterosexual HIV Transmission in Botswana," *New England Journal of Medicine* 367, no. 5 (2012): 423–434; R. M. Grant, J. R. Lama, P. L. Anderson, et al., "Preexposure Chemoprophylaxis for HIV Prevention in Men Who Have Sex with Men," *New England Journal of Medicine* 363, no. 27 (2010): 2587–2599; J. M. Baeten, D. Donnell, P. Ndase, et al., "Antiretroviral Prophylaxis for HIV Prevention in Heterosexual Men and Women," *New England Journal of Medicine* 367, no. 5 (2012): 399–410.

7. L. Van Damme, A. Corneli, K. Ahmed, and K. Agot, "Preexposure Prophylaxis for HIV Infection among African Women," *New England Journal of Medicine* 367, no. 5 (2012): 411–422; J. M. Marrazzo, G. Ramjee, G. Nair, and T. Palanee, "Pre-exposure Prophylaxis for HIV in Women: Daily Oral Tenofovir, Oral Tenofovir/Emtricitabine or Vaginal Tenofovir Gel in the VOICE Study (MTN 003)," 20th Conference on Retroviruses and Opportunistic Infections, Atlanta, 2013.

8. K. R. Amico, M. Wallace, L.-G. Bekker, et al., "Experiences with HPTN 067/ADAPT Study-Provided Open-Label PrEP among Women in Cape

Town: Facilitators and Barriers within a Mutuality Framework," *AIDS and Behavior* (2016): 1–15.

9. A. Burgener and N. Klatt, "Uncovering the Role of the Vaginal Microbiome in Undermining PrEP Efficacy in Women," 21st International AIDS Conference, Durban, 2016.

10. A. Kagee, R. H. Remien, A. Berkman, S. Hoffman, L. Campos, and L. Swartz, "Structural Barriers to ART Adherence in Southern Africa: Challenges and Potential Ways Forward," *Global Public Health* 6, no. 1 (2011): 83–97; B. D. Adam, "Epistemic Fault Lines in Biomedical and Social Approaches to HIV Prevention," *Journal of the International AIDS Society* 14, suppl. 2 (2011): S2.

11. Baeten et al., "Antiretroviral Prophylaxis for HIV Prevention in Heterosexual Men and Women."

12. P. Farmer, M. Connors, and J. Simmons, eds., *Women, Poverty and AIDS: Sex, Drugs and Structural Violence*, 2nd ed. (Monroe, ME: Common Courage Press, 2007).

13. B. D. Adam, "Infectious Behaviour: Imputing Subjectivity to HIV Transmission," *Social Theory and Health* 4, no. 2 (2006): 168–179; A. Gibbs, S. Willan, A. Misselhorn, and J. Mangoma, "Combined Structural Interventions for Gender Equality and Livelihood Security: A Critical Review of the Evidence from Southern and Eastern Africa and the Implications for Young People," *Journal of the International AIDS Society* 15, suppl. 1 (2012): 17362.

14. B. Hanna and A. Kleinman, "Unpacking Global Health," in *Reimagining Global Health: An Introduction*, ed. P. Farmer, J. Y. Kim, A. Kleinman, and M. Basilico (Berkeley: University of California Press, 2013), 15–32.

15. L. Miles, "Women, AIDS, Power and Heterosexual Negotiation: A Discourse Analysis," *Agenda* 15 (1992): 14–28.

16. J. M. Baeten, T. Palanee-Phillips, E. R. Brown, et al., "Use of a Vaginal Ring Containing Dapivirine for HIV-1 Prevention in Women," *New England Journal of Medicine* 375, no. 22 (2016): 2121–2132.

17. A. Nel, N. van Niekerk, S. Kapiga, et al., "Safety and Efficacy of a Dapivirine Vaginal Ring for HIV Prevention in Women," *New England Journal of Medicine* 375, no. 22 (2016): 2133–2143.

18. E. T. Richardson, "Research on Oral Pre-Exposure Prophylaxis in Sub-Saharan Africa Is an Example of Biomedical Tunnel Vision," *AIDS* 28, no. 10 (2014): 1537–1538.

19. Van Damme et al., "Preexposure Prophylaxis for HIV Infection among African Women"; Marrazzo et al., "Pre-exposure Prophylaxis for HIV in Women"; Q. Abdool Karim, S. S. Abdool Karim, J. A. Frohlich, et al., "Effectiveness and Safety of Tenofovir Gel, an Antiretroviral Microbicide, for the Prevention of HIV Infection in Women," *Science* 329, no. 5996 (2010): 1168–1174.

20. M.-C. Boily, R. F. Baggaley, L. Wang, et al., "Heterosexual Risk of HIV-1 Infection per Sexual Act: Systematic Review and Meta-analysis of Observational Studies," *Lancet Infectious Diseases* 9, no. 2 (2009): 118–129.

21. O. Shisana, T. Rehle, L. Simbayi, et al., *South African National HIV Prevalence, Incidence, and Behaviour Survey, 2012* (Cape Town: HSRC Press, 2014); W. Delva, F. Meng, R. Beauclair, et al., "Coital Frequency and Condom Use in Monogamous and Concurrent Sexual Relationships in Cape Town, South Africa," *Journal of the International AIDS Society* 16 (2013): 18034; Statistics South Africa, "Mortality and Causes of Death in South Africa, 2014: Findings from Death Notification," 2014, http://www.statssa.gov.za/publications/P03093/P030932014.pdf.

22. P. N. Krivitsky and M. S. Handcock, "A Separable Model for Dynamic Networks," *Journal of the Royal Statistical Society: Series B (Statistical Methodology)* 76, no. 1 (2014): 29–46; P. N. Krivitsky and S. M. Goodreau, "STERGM—Separable Temporal ERGMs for Modeling Discrete Relational Dynamics with Statnet," 2012, 1–31 https://statnet.csde.washington.edu/trac/raw-attachment/wiki/Resources/STERGMtutorial.pdf.

23. S. Jenness, S. M. Goodreau, and M. Morris, "EpiModel: An R Package for Mathematical Modeling of Infectious Disease over Networks," *Journal of Statistical Software* 84, no. 8 (2018): 1–47.

24. Marrazzo et al., "Pre-exposure Prophylaxis for HIV in Women."

25. Delva et al., "Coital Frequency and Condom Use in Monogamous and Concurrent Sexual Relationships in Cape Town, South Africa."

26. Marrazzo et al., "Pre-exposure Prophylaxis for HIV in Women."

27. S. Cassels and S. M. Goodreau, "Interaction of Mathematical Modeling and Social and Behavioral HIV/AIDS Research," *Current Opinion in HIV and AIDS* 6 (2011): 119–123; S. Cassels, S. J. Clark, and M. Morris, "Mathematical Models for HIV Transmission Dynamics: Tools for Social and Behavioral Science Research," *Journal of Acquired Immune Deficiency Syndromes* 47, suppl. 1 (2008): S34–S39.

28. I. Kohler-Hausmann, "Eddie Murphy and the Dangers of Counterfactual Causal Thinking about Detecting Racial Discrimination," *Northwestern University Law Review* 113, no. 5 (2019): 1163–227; L. Hu, "Disparate Causes, pts. I & II," *Phenomenal World* 2019, available at https://phenomenalworld.org/analysis/disparate-causes-i.

29. S. Schwartz, S. J. Prins, U. B. Campbell, and N. M. Gatto, "Is the 'Well-Defined Intervention Assumption' Politically Conservative?," *Social Science and Medicine* 166 (2016): 254–257.

Pre-Appendices

1. G. E. E. Marcus and M. M. J. Fischer, *Anthropology as Cultural Critique: An Experimental Moment in the Human Sciences* (Chicago: University of Chicago Press, 1999); R. Rottenburg, *Far-Fetched Facts: A Parable of Development Aid* (Cambridge, MA: MIT Press, 2009).

2. S. J. Ndlovu-Gatsheni, *Empire, Global Coloniality and African Subjectivity* (New York: Berghahn, 2013).

3. L. T. Smith, *Decolonizing Methodologies: Research and Indigenous Peoples* (London: Zed Books, 2012).

4. Ndlovu-Gatsheni, *Empire, Global Coloniality and African Subjectivity*.

5. I. M. Young, *Responsibility for Justice* (Oxford: Oxford University Press, 2011).

6. C. W. Mills, "White Ignorance," in *Race and Epistemologies of Ignorance*, ed. S. Sullivan and N. Tuana (Albany: State University of New York Press, 2007), 11–38.

7. J. M. Metzl and H. Hansen, "Structural Competency: Theorizing a New Medical Engagement with Stigma and Inequality," *Social Science and Medicine* 103 (2014): 126–133.

8. A. Mbembe, *Critique of Black Reason* (Durham: Duke University Press, 2017).

9. N. Fraser, *Unruly Practices: Power, Discourse, and Gender in Contemporary Social Theory* (Minneapolis: University of Minnesota Press, 1989).

10. T. Pogge, "Moral Universalism and Global Economic Justice," *Politics, Philosophy and Economics* 1, no. 1 (2002): 29–58.

11. F. Fanon, *Black Skin, White Masks* (Boston: Grove Press, 1967).

12. Wikipedia.org, "Yaguine Koita and Fodé Tounkara," 2018, https://en.wikipedia.org/wiki/Yaguine_Koita_and_Fodé_Tounkara.

13. Mbembe, *Critique of Black Reason*.

14. A. Giridharadas, *Winners Take All: The Elite Charade of Changing the World* (New York: Knopf; 2018).

15. P. Bourgois and J. Schonberg, *Righteous Dopefiend* (Berkeley: University of California Press, 2009); I. Hacking, "Making Up People," in *The Science Studies Reader*, ed. M. Biagioli (New York: Routledge, 1999), 161–171.

16. T. C. Quinn, M. J. Wawer, N. Sewankambo, et al., "Viral Load and Heterosexual Transmission of Human Immunodeficiency Virus Type 1," *New England Journal of Medicine* 342, no. 13 (2000): 921–929.

17. See Angell and Farmer for more in-depth discussions: P. E. Farmer, "Social Medicine and the Challenge of Biosocial Research," in *Partner to the Poor: A Paul Farmer Reader*, ed. H. Saussy (Berkeley: University of California Press, 2010), 248–266; M. Angell, "Investigators' Responsibilities for Human Subjects in Developing Countries," *New England Journal of Medicine* 342, no. 13 (2000): 967–969.

18. R. Gray, G. Kigozi, X. Kong, et al., "The Effectiveness of Male Circumcision for HIV Prevention and Effects on Risk Behaviors in a Posttrial Follow-Up Study," *AIDS* 26, no. 5 (2012): 609–615.

Conclusion

1. M. Bakhtin, *The Dialogic Imagination: Four Essays* (Austin: University of Texas Press, 1981).

2. B. Latour, *Science in Action* (Cambridge, MA: Harvard University Press, 1988).

3. R. Grosfoguel, "Decolonizing Post-Colonial Studies and Paradigms of Political-Economy: Transmodernity, Decolonial Thinking, and Global Coloniality," *Transmodernity* 1, no. 1 (2011).

4. D. Neiwert, *Alt-America: The Rise of the Radical Right in the Age of Trump* (London: Verso, 2017).

5. R. Wilson Gilmore, "Abolition Geography and the Problem of Innocence," in *Futures of Black Radicalism*, ed. G. T. Johnson and A. Lubin (London: Verso, 2003).

6. B. E. Richie, *Arrested Justice: Black Women, Violence, and America's Prison Nation* (New York: NYU Press, 2012).

7. M. Mandel, *How America Gets Away with Murder: Illegal Wars, Collateral Damage and Crimes Against Humanity* (London: Pluto, 2004).

8. J. Y. Kim, J. V. Millen, A. Irwin, and J. Gershman, eds., *Dying for Growth: Global Inequality and the Health of the Poor* (Monroe, ME: Common Courage Press, 2002).

9. J. Hickel, *The Divide: Global Inequality from Conquest to Free Markets* (New York: W. W. Norton, 2018); T. Burgis, *The Looting Machine: Warlords, Oligarchs, Corporations, Smugglers, and the Theft of Africa's Wealth* (New York: Public Affairs, 2016); D. Harvey, *The New Imperialism* (Oxford: Oxford University Press, 2003).

10. A. Giridharadas, *Winners Take All: The Elite Charade of Changing the World* (New York: Knopf; 2018).

11. M. Dubois, C. Wake, S. Sturridge, and C. Bennett, "The Ebola Response in West Africa: Exposing the Politics and Culture of International Aid," working paper, Humanitarian Policy Group, 2015; A. G. Frank, "The Development of Underdevelopment," *Monthly Review* 18, no. 4 (1966): 17–31.

12. S. G. Reddy, "Economics' Biggest Success Story Is a Cautionary Tale," *Foreign Policy* (2019).

13. M. Bakhtin, *Rabelais and His World* (Bloomington: Indiana University Press, 2009).

14. C. Ake, *Social Science as Imperialism: The Theory of Political Development*, 2nd ed. (Ibadan: Ibadan University Press, 1982); A. Cerón, "Neocolonial Epidemiology: Public Health Practice and the Right to Health in Guatemala," *Medicine Anthropology Theory* 6, no. 1 (2019): 30–54.

15. V. Adams, ed., *Metrics: What Counts in Global Health* (Durham: Duke University Press, 2016); E. W. Said, *Orientalism* (New York: Vintage, 1979).

16. N. Chomsky, "The Responsibility of Intellectuals," *New York Review of Books* (1967); A. Ahmad, *In Theory: Classes, Nations, Literatures* (London: Verso, 1992).

17. R. Levins and R. Lewontin, *The Dialectical Biologist* (Cambridge, MA: Harvard University Press, 1985); T. Pogge, *World Poverty and Human Rights*, 2nd ed. (Cambridge: Polity, 2008); N. Scheper-Hughes, "The Primacy of the Ethical: Propositions for a Militant Anthropology," *Current Anthropology* 36, no. 3 (2010): 409–440.

18. H. L. Dreyfus and P. Rabinow, *Michel Foucault: Beyond Structuralism and Hermeneutics*, 2nd ed. (Chicago: University of Chicago Press, 1983).

19. J. Rehmann, *Theories of Ideology: The Powers of Alienation and Subjection* (Chicago: Haymarket Books, 2014); L. Althusser, "Ideology and Ideological State Apparatuses," in *Lenin and Philosophy and other Essays* (New York: Monthly Review Press, 1971); Grosfoguel, "Decolonizing Post-Colonial Studies and Paradigms of Political-Economy."

20. W. D. Mignolo, "Epistemic Disobedience, Independent Thought and De-Colonial Freedom," *Theory, Culture and Society* 26, no. 7–8 (2009): 1–23.

21. A. Rosenberg, "Economic Theory as Political Philosophy," *Social Science Journal* 36, no. 4 (1999): 575–587; A. J. Levinovits, "The New Astrologers," *Aeon* (April 2016); P. Romer, "Mathiness in the Theory of Economic Growth," *American Economic Review* 105, no. 5 (2015): 89–93.

22. E. T. Richardson, M. P. Fallah, J. D. Kelly, and M. B. Barrie, "The Predicament of Patients with Suspected Ebola—Authors' Reply," *Lancet Global Health* 5, no. 7 (2017): e660–e661; P. Farmer and N. G. Campos, "Rethinking Medical Ethics: A View from Below," *Developing World Bioethics* 4, no. 1 (2004):17–41.

23. P. E. Tetlock, *Expert Political Judgment: How Good Is It? How Can We Know?* (Princeton: Princeton University Press, 2017).

24. T. Asad, ed., *Anthropology and the Colonial Encounter* (Amherst, NY: Humanity Books, 1973).

25. B. Agger, *Critical Social Theories* (Boulder: Paradigm, 2006).

26. J. S. Lansing and J. N. Kremer, "Emergent Properties of Balinese Water Temple Networks: Coadaptation on a Rugged Fitness Landscape," *American Anthropologist* 95, no. 1(1993): 97–114.

27. R. Rorty, "Wittgenstein and the Linguistic Turn," in A. Ahmed, ed., *Wittgenstein's Philosophical Investigations: A Critical Guide* (Cambridge: Cambridge University Press, 2010), 129–144, doi:10.1017/ CBO9780511750939.008.

28. D. Graeber, *Fragments of an Anarchist Anthropology* (Chicago: Prickly Paradigm Press, 2004); A. Querejazu, "Encountering the Pluriverse: Looking for Alternatives in Other Worlds," *Revista Brasileira de Política Internacional* 59, no. 2 (2016): e007; R. Rorty, "Solidarity or Objectivity?," in *Relativism: Interpretation and Confrontation*, ed. M. Krausz (Notre Dame: University of Notre Dame Press, 1989), 167–183; https://www .newframe.com/archive-communalist-palaver/.

29. E. Husserl, *The Crisis of European Sciences and Transcendental Phenomenology* (Evanston: Northwestern University Press, 1970).

30. K. Kuhn, "Global Warming and Leishmaniasis in Italy," *Bulletin of Tropical Medicine and International Health* 7, no. 2(1999): 1–2.

31. F. Nietzsche, *The Portable Nietzsche* (New York: Penguin, 1977).

32. A. Mbembe, "What Is Postcolonial Thinking?," *Esprit* (December 2006).

33. Ahmad, *In Theory*.

34. E. T. Richardson and A. Polyakova, "The Illusion of Scientific Objectivity and the Death of the Investigator," *European Journal of Clinical Investigation* 42, no. 2 (2012): 213–215; D. Swartz, *Culture and Power: The Sociology of Pierre Bourdieu* (Chicago: University of Chicago Press, 1997); P. Bourdieu and L. I. D. Wacquant, *An Invitation to Reflexive Sociology* (Chicago: University of Chicago Press, 1992).

35. P. Vannini, "Critical Pragmatism," in L. M. Given, ed., *The Sage Encyclopedia of Qualitative Research Methods* (Thousand Oaks, CA: SAGE Publications, 2008): 160–164.

36. Pogge, *World Poverty and Human Rights*; B. Good, *Medicine, Rationality and Experience: An Anthropological Perspective* (Cambridge: Cambridge University Press, 1994); A. Kleinman, "An Anthropological Perspective on Objectivity: Observation, Categorization, and the Assessment of Suffering," in *Health and Social Change in International Perspective*, ed. L. C. Chen, A. Kleinman, and N. Ware (Cambridge, MA: Harvard University Press, 1994), 129–138.

Part II

1. Z. Bauman, *Liquid Modernity* (Cambridge: Polity, 2000).

Afterword

1. Adapted from E. T. Richardson, "Pandemicity, COVID-19 and the Limits of Public Health 'Science,'" *BMJ Global Health* 5, no. 4 (2020):

e002571; and E. T. Richardson, M. M. Malik, W. A. Darity Jr., A. K. Mullen, M. Malik, M. T. Bassett, P. E. Farmer, L. Worden, and J. H. Jones, "Reparations for Black American Descendants of Persons Enslaved in the U.S. and Their Estimated Impact on SARS-CoV-2 Transmission" (2020), medRxiv 2020.06.04.20112011.

2. Merriam-Webster, "'Pandemic' vs 'Epidemic,'" https://www.merriam-webster.com/words-at-play/epidemic-vs-pandemic-difference (accessed March 27, 2020).

3. M. S. Green, "Did the Hesitancy in Declaring COVID-19 a Pandemic Reflect a Need to Redefine the Term?," *Lancet* 395 (2020): 1034–1035.

4. V. Adams, ed., *Metrics: What Counts in Global Health* (Durham: Duke University Press, 2016).

5. S. L. Dalglish, "COVID-19 Gives the Lie to Global Health Expertise," *Lancet*, published online March 27, 2020, doi:10.1016/S0140-6736(20)30739-X.

6. P. Nadella, A. Swaminathan, and S. V. Subramanian, "Forecasting Efforts from Prior Epidemics and COVID-19 Predictions," *European Journal of Epidemiology* (2020), https://doi.org/10.1007/.s10654-020-00661-0.

7. A. Sayburn, "Covid-19: Experts Question Analysis Suggesting Half UK Population Has Been Infected," *BMJ* 368 (2020), https://www.bmj.com/content/368/bmj.m1216.

8. M. Enserink and K. Kupferschmidt, "Mathematics of Life and Death: How Disease Models Shape National Shutdowns and Other Pandemic Policies," *Science*, published online March 25, 2020, https://www.sciencemag.org/news/2020/03/mathematics-life-and-death-how-disease-models-shape-national-shutdowns-and-other#.

9. E. Bendavid and J. Bhattacharya, "Is the Coronavirus as Deadly as They Say?," *Wall Street Journal*, published online March 24, 2020, https://www.wsj.com/articles/is-the-coronavirus-as-deadly-as-they-say-11585088464.

10. R. Wallace, A. Liebman, L. F. Chaves, and R. Wallace, "COVID-19 and Circuits of Capital," *Monthly Review*, published online March 27, 2020.

11. L. Althusser, "Ideology and Ideological State Apparatuses," in *Lenin and Philosophy and Other Essays* (New York: Monthly Review Press, 1971).

12. E. Bendavid, B. Mulaney, N. Sood, S. Shah, E. Ling, R. Bromley-Dulfano, C. Lai, Z. Weissberg, R. Saavedra-Walker, J. Tedrow, D. Tversky, A. Bogan, T. Kupiec, D. Eichner, R. Gupta, J. Ioannidis, and J. Bhattacharya, "COVID-19 Antibody Seroprevalence in Santa Clara County, California," medRxiv 2020.04.14.20062463.

13. N. P. Jewell, J. A. Lewnard, and B. L. Jewell, "Caution Warranted: Using the Institute for Health Metrics and Evaluation Model for Predicting the Course of the COVID-19 Pandemic," *Annals of Internal Medicine*, published online April 14, 2020, doi:10.7326/M20-1565.

14. P. L. Berger and T. Luckmann, *The Social Construction of Reality: A Treatise in the Sociology of Knowledge* (New York: Anchor, 1967); I. Hacking, *The Social Construction of What?* (Cambridge, MA: Harvard University Press, 1999).

15. M. Foucault, *Discipline and Punish: The Birth of the Prison* (New York: Knopf Doubleday, 1979); E. T. Richardson, M. B. Barrie, J. D. Kelly, Y. Dibba, S. Koedoyoma, and P. E. Farmer, "Biosocial Approaches to the 2013–16 Ebola Pandemic," *Health and Human Rights* 18 (2016): 167–179.

16. D. Graeber, "The Twilight of Vanguardism," in *Possibilities: Essays on Hierarchy, Rebellion, and Desire* (Oakland: AK Press, 2007), 301–311; S. G. Reddy, "Randomise This! On Poor Economics," *Review of Agrarian Studies* 2, no. 2 (2012); C. W. Mills, *The Sociological Imagination* (1959; Oxford: Oxford University Press, 2000).

17. S. Abimbola, "The Foreign Gaze: Authorship in Academic Global Health," *BMJ Global Health* 4, no. 5 (2019): e002068.

18. E. T. Richardson, M. M. Malik, W. A. Darity Jr., A. K. Mullen, M. Malik, M. T. Bassett, P. E. Farmer, L. Worden, and J. H. Jones, "Reparations for Black American Descendants of Persons Enslaved in the U.S.

and Their Estimated Impact on SARS-CoV-2 Transmission" (2020), medRxiv 2020.06.04.20112011.

19. K. Nkrumah, *Neo-colonialism, the Last Stage of Imperialism* (London: Thomas Nelson, 1965).

20. J. Breilh, "Latin American Critical ('Social') Epidemiology: New Settings for an Old Dream," *International Journal of Epidemiology* 37 (2008): 745–750; N. wa Thiong'o, *Decolonising the Mind: The Politics of Language in African Literature* (London: James Curry, 1986); L. T. Smith, *Decolonizing Methodologies: Research and Indigenous Peoples* (London: Zed Books, 2012); R. Muhareb and R. Giacaman, "Tracking COVID-19 Responsibly," *Lancet*, published online March 27, 2020.

21. E. Le Roy Ladurie, *Un concept: L'unification microbienne du monde (XIVe–XVIIe siècles)* (Berne: Société Suisse d'Histoire, 1973); M. H. Green, "The Globalisations of Disease," in N. Boivin, R. Crassard, and M. Petraglia, eds., *Human Dispersal and Species Movement: From Prehistory to the Present* (Cambridge: Cambridge University Press, 2017), 494–520.

22. World Health Organization, "Children: Reducing Mortality," 2019, https://www.who.int/news-room/fact-sheets/detail/children-reducing -mortality (accessed February 4, 2020).

23. P. E. Farmer, *Pathologies of Power: Health, Human Rights, and the New War on the Poor*, 2nd ed. (Berkeley: University of California Press, 2005).

24. I. M. Young, *Responsibility for Justice* (Oxford: Oxford University Press, 2011).

25. E. T. Richardson, M. B. Barrie, J. D. Kelly, Y. Dibba, S. Koedoyoma, and P. E. Farmer, "Biosocial Approaches to the 2013–16 Ebola Pandemic," *Health and Human Rights* 18, no. 1 (2016): 167–179.

Index